BIRTH HAPPENS

BIRTH HAPPENS

A Collection of Birth Stories

Pregnancy is not an illness.
Birth is not an emergency.

Stories collected and edited by
Sarah Beauchamp

For Parker, Elsie, and Quinn

Thank you for making me a mom.
Thank you for lighting up my life.

Introduction

I love everything about pregnancy, birth, and babies. As someone who really struggled with body image issues for most of my life, pregnancy and motherhood made me truly love myself for the first time. Watching my body grow a small person was incredible. Then my body made milk to feed that small human and keep them alive. It was like magic.

I have had three babies and three very different births. I am grateful for the experiences I had because it pushed me to learn more and become educated about what standard prenatal care looks like, especially in America where I live. The more I learned, the angrier I became. The United States has one of the worst maternal mortality rates out of any developed country in the world. We have increasing numbers of inductions and cesarean births, both of which are known to have associated risks and complications.

There is also an increasing amount of birth trauma happening around the globe. Modern research has reported high rates of childbirth trauma in Japan, Turkey, the United Kingdom, and the

United States[1]. It is estimated that up to 40% of first-time birthers may experience trauma during childbirth. Birth trauma can negatively impact breastfeeding and postpartum recovery. It can greatly increase a person's chances of developing a postpartum mood disorder. Birth trauma can also make it hard for new parents to bond with their baby.

Rates of medical interventions are increasing while birth trauma is simultaneously increasing. Rates of medical interventions are increasing while maternal mortality is increasing across Europe and North America. Birthing people deserve better care. It was after learning more about the challenges birthing people face that I was inspired to take a doula certification class and then pursue becoming a licensed midwife. I dream of a system that supports birth without causing harm. Birth trauma is not completely avoidable, but there is so much room for improvement.

The idea for this book came to me after the birth of my third baby. I was also inspired by *Ina May Gaskin's Guide to Childbirth,* which I recommend for any first-time mom to read. In Ina May's book, there is a collection of birth stories from women who gave birth in the 1970's and 80's under the care of midwives in a small community in Tennessee. I wanted to make a more modern collection of birth stories and include stories from around the world. I wanted to create a collection of stories that would be more relatable to people giving birth today.

This collection is all stories from women who gave birth in 2021. You will read about home births, hospital births, and birth center births. You will read about unassisted births and births attended by obstetricians and midwives. You will read about twin births and breech births. You will read about beautiful and powerful births. You will also read about some beautiful but sad births.

One of my dreams for this book is to help destigmatize birth. Birth doesn't have to be scary. It can be enjoyable and even fun! I also hope this book can provide education about the physiology of birth and the options that come with it. I hope *Birth Happens* can help people confidently plan for the birth they want. When you are pregnant, you get to choose who you see for prenatal care, where you want to give birth, and the team that will support you on your birthing day. These decisions are so important and will impact how your birth plays out.

I am forever grateful for all of the amazing women who shared their stories with me to create this resource. I hope these stories provide inspiration and education for anyone who decides to read them.

1 Beck CT, Watson S, Gable RK. Traumatic Childbirth and Its Aftermath: Is There Anything Positive? J Perinat Educ. 2018 Jun;27(3):175-184. doi: 10.1891/1058-1243.27.3.175. PMID: 30364308; PMCID: PMC6193358.

January

January 5, 2021

Sonya and Elsie: A Birth in Arizona

She always felt different. She felt fierce and ready. Somehow I knew she would come earlier than the guess date. Still, those labor pains 15 days early came as a surprise. I rocked and swayed in the shower thinking it wasn't actually happening. Around 1:00am I woke up Rusty and we decided to meet up with my midwife, Alyssa, to check my dilation. At the early morning check I was 4 centimeters dilated. Rusty and I were elated. My midwife was a bit surprised at our excitement, but with our first, even after over thirty hours of labor, I never dilated past 3 centimeters.

We were so unprepared for Elsie's arrival. I headed home to finish laundry before we headed to our assistant midwife, Lisette's home. I'm forever grateful for her invitation to birth in her home, as our home wasn't an option. When we arrived, Alyssa and Lisette welcomed us. As we found our groove, things began to progress fast, fast enough that we weren't sure we would have time to fill the birth tub. The care I received is beyond words. To be loved and cared for without judgment of grunts, groans, roars, tears and laughter... it's incredibly humbling and empowering.

In preparation for Elsie's birth, I tried to connect with her and visualize labor and delivery. The ONLY clear thing that ever came was a vivid and powerful image of looking at her and being bathed in early sunrise rays. As our birthing room filled with bright morning light and she wasn't in my arms, I knew something was off, but I didn't want to believe it.

Soon enough, the midwife realized I was fighting against a cervical lip. I was progressing, but a portion of my cervix was still blocking the exit. My body was wanting to push, but Elsie had nowhere to really go. We decided to have Alyssa manually try to hold the lip out of the way during a contraction. This was the only time I felt PAIN. Natural labor pain is different from what I felt during those contractions. After a few rounds of pain, we decided we would just let my body dissolve my cervix on its own. Eventually I just wanted to shut my eyes and nap. So I did just that. I distinctly remember hearing Rusty's voice change and him yelling for the midwife to come back in the room.

I heard them all tell me to wake up and call my name. I couldn't figure out why they were all around me. I heard something about smelling salts. "Try again." "Peppermint oil." "Salts again." I was so confused when I came to in the middle of a full-blown contraction with peppermint oil on my nose. My nap was actually a loss of consciousness. Rusty later told me he felt totally helpless as I slumped over in his arms. My midwife checked both the baby's and my vitals - both were perfect. We were all a bit perplexed by the whole situation. My midwife looked at me and I knew what she was about to say before the words hit the air. Transfer. We agreed this was out of the range of normal, and although I desperately wanted to avoid a transfer, we needed to. She let me mourn my change of plans and I gave her the nod to call 911.

It's the oddest feeling hearing sirens and knowing they are for you. After multiple IV pokes, temperature checks, and asking if the baby was crowning, I laid there on the floor trying to figure out what insurance would cover for the ambulance. A firefighter asked if any amount of money was worth my life. I laughed and said, "Well maybe." He wasn't sure what to do with that. The midwife and I tried one last hail Mary attempt to manually hold the cervical lip out of the way so Elsie could just pop out, but it was to no avail.

In the ambulance, I heard a firefighter ask for a scalpel. I yelled, "For what?!"

He said, "Uhm, the umbilical cord?"

Rusty yelled from the front cab, "There's a baby?!?"

I grabbed the paramedic by her shirt and firmly said, "DO NOT LET HIM TOUCH THE CORD!"

The firefighter finally gave in and asked, "Ma'am, do you want to just hold my hand?"

"Yes. Thank you."

Soon enough we rolled through the back entrance. I remember laughing and telling myself to let it go and lean into the unwanted transfer. Once in the labor and delivery room, they quickly transferred me off the plastic tarp with my broken waters onto a dry bed. I immediately turned myself around and onto my knees. The attending OB walked in, announced who he was, and continued to the back out of the room. As he walked, he mumbled something including "c-section" and "forceps."

At this point any calm and positivity I had mustered up instantly dissipated. I began screaming for Rusty, who was behind the curtain trying to sort out paperwork to get Lisette allowed in the room. Rusty came around the curtain and I yelled about the doctor saying c-section. My husband is a man full of a calm and caring energy. Yet on this day, some type of Papa Bear turned on.

Suddenly, I heard his and the doctor's voices rising with intensity. I looked between my legs to see Rusty and the doctor literally chest to chest like two gorillas. Lisette knew the doctor and knew my husband and stepped in as referee, calming them both down. I laughed. I was just so over it all. The commotion, the sound, the heat, the intense pressure, and the crazy desire to... poop. I switched my focus from baby to simply pooping. Rusty told me it was the tiniest turd he'd ever seen, but it was enough to relieve the pressure it was creating.

I put one hand on my belly, the other on the bed. I closed my eyes and made everything else in the room disappear but Elsie and me. I thought, "Okay, baby girl. Next one. You ready?" When the next contraction came, I welcomed it with my whole being. I literally felt the cervical lip give way and Elsie flew out. I instinctively caught her. I pulled her to me. There is absolutely nothing to prepare you for the joy, the quiet, the surprise, the relief. The whole moment you catch your baby and lay eyes on the little human you felt grow within you.

As we situated ourselves, I felt my placenta deliver and more gushes. From looking at Rusty's face and hearing the doctor explaining Pitocin, I knew I was hemorrhaging. It was stopped and I am forever grateful no more interventions were needed. We settled into our room and my husband went home to be with our older daughter, while I spent some one-on-one time with Elsie. I held her, confused at her arrival into a noisy busy room, filled with harsh bright lights. So opposite from what I had seen and felt.

The next morning, I opened my tired, tear-poofed eyes to exactly the vision I had before with all the details filled in. Sunrise rays filled the room, bathing us both in light. I *knew* I didn't fail. We had done it together. Seeing her there in the warmth of the morning glow, I knew it had all happened as it was meant to. We were supported by an incredible partner and team.

When people ask about Elsie's birth, I think of the immense laughter we had with my team during labor. I think of the genuine care I received. I think of the tender moments that words cannot convey. Birth will never cease to amaze me. I am stronger, more empowered, different, and better after having gone through what I did. I will forever advocate for choice and for a powerful birth team to surround you. Thank you, Elsie, for choosing me to be your mama and making your birth your own.

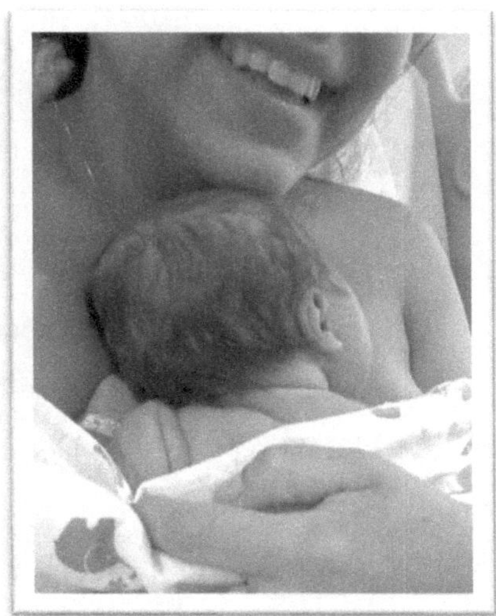

Kelcey and Noah: A Birth in Oklahoma

I woke around 4:00am with the first surges. After a strong one I thought, "What have I done? I could have had pain medicine for this!" As it passed, I reminded myself of the affirmations I had prepared and felt better. I had all these ideas for things I would do during early labor, but all I could do was lay there and breathe. I turned on my hypnobirthing app and started timing surges.

Around noon we called the birth center to tell them what was going on. We had an appointment already scheduled for that afternoon, and the midwife told us to just come in then. The birth center was 45 minutes away, but the ride seemed to go quite fast. I kept the app with the relaxing meditations going, and I breathed to get through surges. We arrived at 2:00pm and I consented to a cervical check. I was 3 centimeters dilated and 100% effaced. They let us stay since we lived so far away.

We settled into a large room with natural light, a cozy bed, and a big tub. It was so beautiful and relaxing. At 3:00 they checked me again and I was at 9 centimeters! I was so happy, I thought it was almost over. The midwife said, "Let's have this baby!" I got into the tub and the surges mellowed out. My husband and I were left alone for a while, it may have been a couple of hours, and the midwives came in periodically to check on us. The baby's heartbeat was always steady and strong. I was stuck at 9 centimeters with a cervical lip in the way. The midwife held the lip out of the way during a couple of contractions, and finally I was at a 10.

I can't say I really felt the urge to push, but the surges were so strong I didn't know what to do. Pushing felt better than not pushing, so I went with it. The tub was getting uncomfortable, and it was too slippery to get traction, so we went to the bed. I laid on my back with one foot on each midwives' shoulders and my husband at my side. I thought anytime they would be saying they could see the baby's head. I pushed for 1.5 hours. I had no idea I could push that hard. I thought my body would just do it. I had heard about the fetal ejection reflex and was expecting that to do the job, but it did not.

I pushed with every ounce of my being. I pushed so hard I couldn't help but release the loudest bloodcurdling primal scream that had ever left my body. I pushed so hard I could feel the pressure move up my body like a heat wave from my vagina to my face and out the top of my head. I pushed for hours, for days, for eternity. I was outside of time. I would push for the rest of my life.

Finally, the midwife told me to reach down and feel the head. I didn't want to, I don't know why, so she took my hand and put it there for me. I'm so glad she did. I could only feel the tiniest patch of soft hair, but it was enough to keep me going and help me push even harder. After feeling the head, I really thought it was almost done, surely there couldn't be more than two or three surges left. A little while later I felt the head again, and the squishy patch of hair had grown just a little bit bigger. The midwife said it was going perfectly, she wouldn't want it to go any faster than this. I was reassured. I didn't want to tear and had prepared myself to go slowly while he was crowning. In the moment it was hard, I just wanted it to be over!

Between surges I have never been more relaxed. Every muscle in my face - my jaw, eyebrows, the space behind my eyes - was without tension. Finally, the midwives told my husband to go catch the baby, and I knew it was almost finished. The baby crowned and it stung like fire. He finally popped out in a sweet release of warm and wet. He was placed on my chest so abruptly. I was savoring that sweet gush, that emptiness between my legs, and it was really a shock to remember what it was all for! He cried a bit and then pulled his head up to see us, eyes full of wonder. The placenta came within minutes, and we had our golden hour. It was perfect. I am eternally grateful to my husband, Sean, and the wonderful midwives Hannah, Crystal, and Gail for their support!

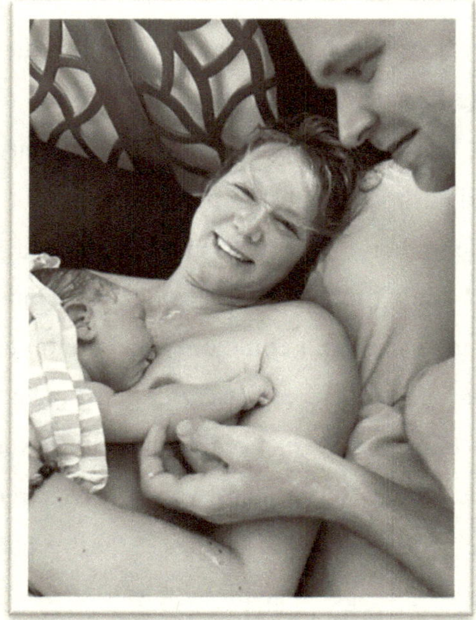

January 20, 2021

Devon and Finn

I had been dealing with prodromal labor for two weeks at this point and it was the day after my due date. I never made it to my due date with my first baby, so this was new territory for me. I went in for my 40-week midwife appointment and I was 2.5 centimeters dilated. My contractions seemed to be getting closer together. Our fourth wedding anniversary was the next day, so my husband and I decided to go play mini golf to celebrate because it was close to home if my labor started getting too intense. As we were playing, I started having some pretty intense contractions, but I was determined to finish the game because I was winning. I won and the contractions tapered off. Around 10:00pm on the 19th my contractions were about 4 minutes apart and lasting 90 seconds. I work at a home birth/birth center and my boss was my midwife. I contacted her and she said I could decide when I wanted to head to the birth center. I waited another hour just to make sure my contractions stayed strong and consistent.

I labored at the birth center for a long time and around 2:00am the contractions stalled. I went back home around 8:00. All day on the 20th I had lots of contractions, but they would stall and were not consistent. I was soaking up the potential last day as a family of three. My parents picked up my almost 2-year-old so we could get some rest and focus on laboring. Around 4:00pm my contractions were getting super intense and turning into back labor, so I got in the tub to help soothe my back pain. I had back labor with my first and I knew the familiar feeling and could tell my baby boy would arrive soon. A coworker texted to check on me and see if I needed anything - sprite, chocolate milkshake and raspberries was my request. My coworker arrived and saw that I was deep into labor land and checked with my husband, who was pouring water down my back, that the midwife had been called --which she had. At 5:00pm the midwife arrived and checked my progress ---I was only 3 centimeters dilated with a high cervical lip! I was so disappointed and exhausted. I was losing hope that I could do this unmedicated because it was so intense, my contractions were so close together, and I had barely made any progress in the last 24 hours. She offered to stretch my cervix during a contraction to see if she could get it to dilate more. She was such a saint and held my cervix with every contraction for FIVE HOURS! She tried to let go at one point and I asked her...well more like said, "Don't take your hand off..."

At 10:00pm I started having the urge to push and pushed until 10:50 when I could finally feel my baby's hairy head. At 11:00 my baby boy Finn was born! My labor with my first was such a stark contrast and this was a shock for a second birth. Looking back, I didn't think it would ever end but it made me a stronger woman because of how I handled it and pushed through to have the home birth I dreamed of. I couldn't have done it without the amazing support and hours upon hours of counterpressure from my husband, my coworker who brought snacks and encouragement, and my midwife for her heart, compassion and strength to get my son here. While it wasn't a fast labor like I had hoped for, it was what I needed to prove how strong I really am. We also have a pretty cute anniversary gift.

January 28, 2021

Deserea and Andreiel

My son was born at 10:53pm on January 28th. Contractions started around 4:00am that day and went on all day. I did a bit of bouncing on an exercise ball as well as a lot of walking and stair climbing once I realized I was definitely in labor. I stayed home as long as I possibly could and timed my contractions to the point where I felt it was necessary to go to the hospital.

I left for the hospital around 6:00pm. Once I got there my labor began to stall a bit. I think it happened because I stopped moving as much as I was at home and stopped really focusing on getting through every contraction. Being at the hospital brought lots of distractions into my labor. When I had a cervical check, I was 8 centimeters dilated. My dilation didn't change until about an hour before my son was born. I had a birth plan that the hospital thankfully followed. The nurses I had were pretty patient with my labor for the most part. I was offered Pitocin to try and speed things up, but I declined. I was also asked if I wanted them to break my water, but I declined that as well. I am thankful they respected my decisions and didn't push interventions on me. Even when I almost gave in, they didn't pressure me and still left the decisions up to me.

Overall, my birth experience was a blessed one, I am thankful for how it turned out and only wish I would've educated myself a bit more before I went to the hospital!

February

February 3, 2021

Emily and Joanna: A Birth in Virginia

The birth of my daughter was everything it wasn't supposed to be. It was the exact opposite of what I had planned. The day and moment I became a mother was the loss of a moment I will never get back.

My daughter is my first baby. For 9 months I had my heart set on a homebirth. I was quick in finding a midwife I loved and trusted. For months I read through piles of books and binged on podcasts. I could not wait to be the birthing mother in all the videos I watched. I was going to catch my baby and feel an amazing sense of pride in what my body had done. Everything about my pregnancy was healthy, normal, and should have been predictable. Only in the last hour before she was born did it fall apart.

After months of anticipation, "baby day" finally came. My body was ready, and labor began with consistent contractions around 6:00pm. My husband and I didn't even go to bed that night. We cleaned the house top to bottom, with brief pauses here and there as the intensity built. We called and updated my midwives around

1:00am. When they arrived at 3:00, I was measuring about 6 centimeters dilated. A few more hours of intense contractions went by. Everyone was doing their best to keep me comfortable. I sat in the tub, laid on the bed, spent time on the floor, and sat on the birth ball. It was lots of moving and passing time. My water broke with a gush around 9:00am. That's when the pushing began. Hard and intense, my body went on for two hours. I was still making progress but was absolutely exhausted. After the last cervical check, my midwife calmly informed us that my baby was in a surprise breech position, and because she was not certified to deliver, we would be transferring to the hospital. Fast forward less than 45 minutes later, and Joanna Kate was born via C-section under general anesthesia.

I lost so many things that day. Even if she is healthy. Even if I am healthy. Even if c-sections are valid births. Even with all these things, it is still a loss I grieve. I was asleep when my baby was born. My husband met her without me. I didn't want to hold her when I woke up. I was in so much groggy pain. I felt alone. We waited to find out the gender, and that moment was taken away when I heard "it's a girl" before becoming coherent. The first two weeks of recovery involved a uterine infection and re-admission to the hospital. It took weeks before I was able to enjoy my baby and take care of her. So much loss. Disappointment. Anger. Jealousy. The first year postpartum was a never-ending snowball of hard emotions to sort through.

I can share the facts of my birth easily. I love birth! I am a huge believer and advocate for natural, low- intervention, birth! But how to handle the trauma of the broken system I have experienced firsthand; a system that would rather perform major abdominal surgery before training breech certified midwives. That is a harder thing to talk about. My only combat to what I lost, is choosing to see what I have, and didn't know to look forward to it. I clung to the "nothing like the moment that baby lays on your chest for the first time". I desperately anticipated that experience, and never got it. I try to be hopeful for next time, but it doesn't heal the hurt now.

My coping method has been to replace the narrative everyday with, "Nothing like the moment…your baby smiles at you for the first time, giggles, or gives you a hug. The moment she blows you a kiss. Splashes in the tub. Cries when you leave. Feeds you her snack. Takes her first steps. Falls asleep in your arms. Crawls into your lap with a book."

Motherhood is made up of LOTS of beautiful moments. Birth trauma has made me try harder to see and appreciate them.

February 4, 2021

Jori and Remington

It all started Tuesday morning. I was 41 weeks pregnant. I had spent the last almost ten months preparing and envisioning Remi's birth. We had everything ready. We were ready, but nothing was happening yet. As a birth worker, I know it's normal to go past your due date. But as a new mom, I was anxious and wanted to get things going. Nancy came over to check in on us for our regular weekly visit and I asked her to check me. Nancy made the comment that she couldn't remember the last time she checked someone prior to labor, but it was what I wanted. Matt and I made the decision that if I was dilated enough, we'd do a membrane sweep.

I responded really well to the sweep and Nancy reminded me that this could kick me into labor, but it could also cause false labor. She went home and Matt went to work. I laid down on the couch and attempted to nap. About two hours after everyone left. I thought I was going into labor. All the normal labor signs... but also, all the normal false labor, post sweep signs. I had bloody show, cramping that turned into contractions, and lost my mucus plug. This all happened over the next 24 hours. I got no sleep. My contractions were every 3-4 minutes. I should have known better... I was coping too well, too talkative, and too happy, but we called the team over anyway because to us, in that moment, THIS was it! I had to be close!

Everyone arrived. It was Wednesday morning, and we were all so excited. Something in me felt like I needed answers about where I was because honestly, I wasn't convinced that this was actually it. I knew what active labor looked like and as excited as we were to be parents, I knew that what I was feeling couldn't be active labor. My contractions were close together, consistent, and palpable, but I was too calm and collected. I couldn't be this great at managing the pain of labor... could I?

Nancy checked me and I had not made any progress. This sucked to hear and our girl was not ready to be born yet. At this point, we sent everyone home and Matt and I were told to relax and sleep. When my contractions stayed 3-4 minutes apart for the next couple hours, and I couldn't sleep, we called Nancy back over so she could administer therapeutic rest. I think I got 2 hours before the contractions kicked back in.

For the next couple hours, I labored side-lying, in the tub, and in the shower. By 7:00pm, I was truly exhausted and I went to lay down in our guest bedroom for a change of scenery. Just as I was falling asleep, my water broke! And not just a trickle, it exploded. Now, it was time!

By 10:00pm, everyone was back to the house, I was in the tub, and I was laboring hard. Things get fuzzy for me around this point, and I lost all track of time. I think from this point on I kept my eyes closed. I was so focused on making it through each wave that in my mind, if I opened my eyes, I wouldn't be able to get focused again.

Matt stepped up in the biggest way I think he's ever stepped up in his life. He got in the trenches with me and actively met me where I needed him to meet me. Nancy, Mallorie, and Nicole encouraged me, hydrated me, and just sat with me in the space that I created. I filled that space with tears, moans, and straight up power. I was moving that baby through my body, and I felt every move she made. I took every wave as it came and rested between each one. I would almost fall completely asleep for the brief moments of nothingness that I had between each wave. And I did that for what felt like the next century. Then... my body started to push for me.

The contractions would build and at the peak, my body naturally bared down. I was starting to push. About every other contraction the pushing would happen, but I wasn't feeling change. We made our way into the bedroom because I couldn't get in a good position in the tub. I tried hands and knees on the bed and hated it. I tried left side-lying and hated it. I tried over the ball in the bed and absolutely hated it. I needed to know where I was. Did I need to prepare for 12 more hours of this or was my baby coming soon? I asked Nancy to check me. We discussed an anterior lip. If it was there, I wanted her to make it be gone. I knew that involved work from me, but I was prepared for that. Sure enough, I was 9.5 centimeters with a small anterior lip. That's all that stood between me and my girl. One big push and I was complete.

I pushed for a little over an hour and then our girl was here! Remington Louise Sessa, 9 pounds 8 ounces and 21 inches long, born at 3:20am on February 4th, at home into her father's hands. She was perfect, the hard part was over, and WE WERE PARENTS! I did it! I birthed my baby at home like I had supported so many women before me to do. We laid in our bed with our baby girl surrounded by the most incredible people who helped me safely welcome our girl earth side. It was pure magic

Shortly after delivering my placenta, Nancy was inspecting it to make sure it was complete. I felt something move through my body and Nancy's face changed. She looked at the "clot" that had just exited my body and her face turned tearful. I knew, in that moment, I knew. The words that came out of my mouth, in disbelief, "Is it a twin?" Nancy nodded her head yes. She showed me the perfect remains of about a 12–15 week-old fetus. I was pregnant with twins. Matt and I had joked for months in the beginning of my pregnancy about being pregnant with twins and how we would have been ok had we been blessed with that. It didn't feel so funny now.

This beautiful moment of welcoming our daughter earth side was rocked by another sweet babe who didn't make it. I'll be honest, I still think about HER often. We had testing performed on our sweet babe and we were pregnant with twin girls. Would she have looked like Remi? How would I have done two? Would they both look like Matt? Would she have favored me more? Why didn't she make it? Was it my fault? How did we never hear her heartbeat or see her on an ultrasound? For whatever reason, she didn't survive, but I did carry her into this world. My body preserved her alongside her sister for almost ten months and I will always be their mother.

To the sweet girl I didn't get to meet, I love you dearly and can't wait to meet you one day.

February 7, 2021

Alexandria and Adalee

On February 5th I went into my midwife's office to do a membrane sweep around 4:00pm in the afternoon. I was about one centimeter dilated at the time. My husband, Josh, and I went to dinner with his parents a few hours later and I remember feeling very light contractions. Josh and I went home afterwards anticipating that maybe our precious little girl would be born the next day.

We went home and went to bed to get as much sleep as we possibly could before our baby girl arrived. I had a contraction at midnight that was strong enough to wake me, however I knew that it would take a while until the contractions were consistent and close together, so I went back to sleep. I woke a few more times in the next few hours, including around 2:00 and 3:00, after soaking through my underwear. At the time, I thought nothing of it. I guess I was so focused on getting lots of sleep and laboring for as long as I could at home.

Around 6:00am I woke up feeling refreshed, but also with strong enough contractions that I couldn't sleep anymore. I kind of got ready and prepared, pretty convinced that it would be the day. Around 8:00am my contractions were consistently less than seven minutes apart going on almost two hours, but they were not strong. I remember thinking that I would still be in labor for a long time. We decided to call the doctor and ask if we should come in, and he said yes.

I remember telling Josh that I didn't want to go in because I heard that, "Once you get to the hospital, your contractions will go away." Josh told me that we needed to listen to the advice of our doctor. We got all ready, grabbed the bags and made our way! When we got there around 9:00am, they got us all checked in and of course, my contractions seemed to disappear. Just from the timing of my contractions, our nurse had told us that it's not time, but she did ask me a question that led me to tell her about my soaked underwear earlier that morning. She said she wanted to test and make sure it wasn't my water breaking before she sent us home.

She came back and told us that, indeed, my water had broken (partially). There was concern here because I had tested positive for Group B Strep and was told that I needed to be on an antibiotic as soon as, if not before, my water broke because of the increased risk of infection. Since I had already not been on the antibiotic for several hours, they wanted to start me on it right away, so my husband and I were there to stay! The nurse had checked me and I think I was about three centimeters dilated and very effaced.

A few hours went by, and the nurse checked me again and I was still three centimeters dilated. Then another few hours went by, and I was STILL 3 centimeters dilated. The on-call doctor came in, concerned that I was not progressing. He explained that the risk of group B grows as I spend more time in labor and he wanted to speed things along. I was set on as natural of a birth as possible, however, obviously I was concerned about the health of our baby, so I agreed to receive Pitocin around 4:00pm.

Within the hour my contractions were almost intolerable and the nurse had to turn down the Pitocin twice. I was pretty miserable at this point. I couldn't hang on any longer and around 6:00pm, I finally caved and received the epidural. The nurse had checked me again at this point and I was only 5 centimeters dilated. I remember thinking I was so glad I got the epidural. At this point I was so exhausted I don't remember much until around 2:00am on February 7th.

The nurse had come in to check me again and I don't remember how dilated I was, but I do remember her saying that I was close. Very shortly after, I remember feeling a slight pressure, like I had to poop. My husband told the nurse and people started to enter our room left and right. Pushing was the easiest part of my entire labor, it felt like it was only 20 minutes (when I was actually pushing closer to 45 minutes). I did not feel anything other than some pressure. I had a mirror set-up and I could see all of my little girl's hair and then all of the sudden my beautiful baby girl was out and on my chest and it was the best, most indescribable feeling in the entire world.

I heard the doctor mention that I tore more than average, but she stitched me right up while I held my baby girl and I did not feel a thing. Giving birth was absolutely the most incredible and beautiful thing I have and will ever do and I can't wait to have more kids and do it all again. Even though I went in with completely different expectations, I believe everything happened exactly how it was meant to.

February 8, 2021

Kayla and Emilia: A Birth in California

It was a Sunday and I was eight days past my due date. My mom had been staying with us since January 30th, eagerly waiting for my labor to begin so she could meet her granddaughter. My sister had flown in from Washington to be with me while I gave birth. Everyone was so impatient to meet little Emilia, including myself. But today I had decided that whatever happened would happen, and the baby would come when she was ready.

I tried to spend the day doing normal things. My husband and I went to run errands and I spent time with my mom while crocheting the blanket I had started for my daughter. My husband went to bed at

10:00pm because he had to work the next morning. I finished my blanket around 11:00 and went to soak in the bath, my nightly ritual during my third trimester to ease my back and hip pain. While I soaked in the tub, I felt some tightening in my belly. I thought it was just Braxton-Hicks, so I didn't really think anything of it. But then it kept happening and getting stronger. I got my timer app out and started timing them. I was having contractions about 5 minutes apart. They weren't too bad, but I did have to start focusing to get through them.

I drained the tub and got in the shower and labored in there for a while. I kept track and kept breathing through them. Around 2:00am I woke my mom and showed her my app, and she said it looked like I was in labor and that I should go ahead and call my midwife. I called her and let her know my contractions were about 3-4 minutes apart and sent her screenshots of my app. She said it looked like I had progressed pretty far and that I could start heading over to the birth center. I woke my husband and we took our time getting ready to go. We grabbed our go-bag, and we got in the car. The birth center was about 35 minutes away and we arrived around 3:15am.

We got settled in one of the rooms while the midwife and her assistants were setting up the birth pool. She did a cervical check, my first one in pregnancy, and I was already dilated to 6 centimeters! I got in the birth pool, had my husband put on Family Guy, and I just closed my eyes and rode the waves of contractions while listening to the show in the background.

Most of my labor is a blur. I couldn't tell you how long I was in the pool. I know I tried moving around and laboring in different positions. I labored on the toilet; I labored on the bed with a peanut ball. I remember at some point my midwife offered to break my water and I consented. I remember at some point telling my husband I couldn't do this anymore and I wanted to go to the hospital for some pain relief, and he encouraged me and told me I had come so far already and I was almost there. I remember saying that I wasn't ready to be a mom, I couldn't do it, and I was afraid of failing. And I remember my mom, sister, and all the ladies in the room encouraging me and telling me I could do it and I would be a great mother.

At some point a birth stool was offered for me to labor on, so gravity could help get the baby into a better position. I labored on the birth stool for a while. My midwife checked me again and I was fully dilated, the baby was engaged, and if I wanted, I could start pushing. They offered to help me move back into the birth pool. I said, "Nope, I'm too afraid to move. I'm doing this right here."

I sat on the birth stool and my husband sat behind me, giving me support. I was encouraged to listen to my body for when it was time to push. With the next wave, I started to push. I remember just pushing a little bit and then feeling my body push all on its own. It was like throwing up out of my butt. It was such a scary feeling for me, but I knew that I was doing it right. I continued pushing when it felt right and I started to feel the ring of fire. Everyone reminded me to reach down and touch her head, so I did. I felt a head full of hair. I kept pushing with each wave and after about 40 minutes, and a little bit of maneuvering from my midwife due to a stuck shoulder, my daughter Emilia was born at 4:13pm on February 8th.

Every fear and doubt I had melted away when my baby was in my arms. I remember choking up and crying, I remember saying, "Oh my God!" over and over again. I said hello to this precious bundle of joy I had grown in my body, in complete awe of how perfect she was. Her eyes were wide and full of wonder. She looked around the room, so curious about this new world around her. Then she let out a cry. It was the most perfect cry, and I remember feeling overwhelmed with joy. The adrenaline and oxytocin were hitting me full force, and I felt like I could do absolutely anything.

I birthed my placenta shortly afterwards and my husband cut the cord. We spent time bonding together, the three of us, and then she met her grandparents on both sides. My midwife performed the newborn exam, and she was 7 pounds 2 ounces and 19 inches long. I had the slightest upward tear, not even worth suturing. Around 8:30pm, we loaded up in the car to start heading home. I couldn't wait to be home. Home with my new perfect little family.

February 10, 2021
Tabitha and Jane

I've always had varying gestations for my babies, so I knew my fourth baby would be no different. At 37 weeks I began to feel completely worn out by the frequent Braxton Hicks contractions, the heaviness in my pelvis, and the general fatigue from being pregnant while chasing around my three other kids who were six, four, and two. My midwife had determined she was head down and engaged at 34 weeks, which didn't surprise me, but the baby's heaviness definitely did as I'd had small babies in the past.

By late Tuesday night, after cooking a dinner I truly didn't want to cook, I began feeling light contractions. They started about 10 to 12 minutes apart. I avoided telling my husband as I wanted to be sure, and I spent the evening keeping track of them until bedtime when I finally told him they were about seven minutes apart. We watched a show and I fell asleep wondering if it was the real deal. I woke up to more intense contractions around midnight. They'd become five minutes apart and I retreated to our master bathroom to labor on my own, using my birthing ball, leaning on the sink countertop, and lying on the carpet in our closet. Although I knew it was time, I felt sensitive to waking my husband and waited until they were 4 minutes apart before I tentatively woke him up and called the midwife. It was 2:00am and a major ice storm was beginning in the area, so although I had considered waiting longer, with my close contractions and the possibility of worse weather on the way, I let her know to head in my direction.

I continued laboring while my husband prepared the bed and spread out a tarp on our carpet. This was our fourth home birth and he was a pro; it didn't take him long and since I preferred laboring by myself, he settled in the background on his computer. My midwife and her assistant arrived shortly and checked the baby's heart rate. Everything was fine and they went back to the living room to give me space. My other children continued sleeping. With contractions two minutes apart, I labored from 2:00am until 8:00, trying a variety of positions, using my own jet tub, and occasionally trying to catch bits of rest between contractions.

My mother-in-law took our kids out of the house when they woke up and I was worn out. My midwife saw I was beginning to grow tired and suggested a cervical check since my water still hadn't broken. It was the first cervical check I'd had my entire pregnancy and labor. "You're 9 centimeters," she said to my surprise. I'd always had my water broken in the past because my body seemed resistant to breaking it on its own. My midwife advised me to keep squatting. Transition hit not long after and I went on my knees, overpowered by the contractions. My husband and the assistant joined us. I began to shake uncontrollably between contractions and my silence turned into me begging for pressure and massage on my back between contractions.

I tried pushing but still my water wasn't breaking. After half an hour or so, I told the midwife I wanted her to break my water, knowing it could finish the process as it had my other labors. She agreed and then held back a cervical lip with my consent while I pushed. Still kneeling, the baby's head came out and there was a pause. My midwife and assistant were shocked to see her blink, open her eyes, and flash a quick smile as if she was unaffected by birth! With a few more pushes, she came into the world.

Holding her was my dream. A dream of having four babies of mine at home. Different midwives, different houses, but all the same grit, power, love and joy. I am done having more babies, and I am overwhelmed by the blessing it was to have my four.

Welcome to the world, Jane Hope!

February 11, 2021

Jamie and Oliver

I started having prodromal labor at night on Tuesday, February 9th. Contractions started when I laid down to sleep and came regularly every 7 to 8 minutes. They were pretty weak though, and never picked up speed. On Wednesday the contractions were more inconsistent but definitely lasted the entire day. I was feeling "off" that day too, like I was getting sick. I needed to just sit and rest. Along with the contractions, I had major cramps that stayed all day. By 4:00pm I had lost my mucous plug and the contractions started to get more intense. They never seemed to get longer, but it was becoming more difficult to breathe through them without really focusing. I called my mom around 1:00pm and asked her to drive down. She lives about an hour from us, and the anxiety of not knowing when she should come had been weighing on me. Something told me things were progressing.

As she walked in the front door, I remember calling out to her from the bathroom, "I just lost my mucous plug!" We put the kids to bed that night and I stood outside their doors and bawled. I was super emotional. AJ and I attempted to watch some TV, but I felt like crap and went to bed around 9:00. The contractions continued to get more intense. I was having a hard time breathing through them at this point. They were still only 8-10 minutes apart though, so I laid down and tried to rest between them. Finally, around 11:00pm, I told AJ it was time to go. As I looked outside, I was so worried to see it had already started snowing. As we left, he kept saying "I think it's too early to go." And I agreed the contractions were not nearly as close together as I remember with the older kids. I still felt like we should go, though. We stopped once on the way and pulled over because it had been a while since my last contraction, and I was debating going back and waiting at home longer. But the snow was really coming down. The roads were completely covered and I worried we'd end up having a worse drive later if we turned back. AJ was being cautious while driving, but I was terrified. Especially on the bridge over the icy river. I just kept bawling and asking him to drive slower.

At this point I was in active labor and didn't even realize it. Each contraction was longer than a minute and I had to breathe through them. I still was able to have full conversations between contractions, though, so I thought it was still early. When we got to the hospital we had to park and walk a long way to check in. A woman frantically checked us into what looked like a completely empty labor and delivery ward. I kept thinking we were too early and how awful it would be to be sent home.

When we finally made it to the intake room, a sweet midwife named Jamie asked if I'd like to be checked. I agreed, and she said I was 6 centimeters, 100% effaced, and with a bulging bag. When I heard I was 6 centimeters I started bawling tears of joy. It was such a relief to know that my body was working and that we didn't have to go home. This was it!

We moved to a birth room and my contractions immediately started getting stronger. I stood on the floor and leaned my top half on a birth ball I had placed on the bed. AJ left to get our bags from the car for just ten minutes and the nurse went to grab supplies. I remember liking the feeling of being alone for a few minutes to just focus on my breathing. By the time everyone was back, I was ready and begging to get in the tub. After being asked two or three times if we'd like to start an IV, and after really thinking about it (AJ was really helpful to ask for space and time on this), I agreed. She quickly set it up and I hopped in the tub.

The midwife grabbed a cup and spent what felt like forever pouring warm bath water across my belly as I tried to relax and get through each contraction. I was squeezing my hands on the sides of the tub and was losing feeling in them. They'd cramp up to the point where I couldn't move my hands at all. I remember the midwife and AJ massaging my fingers and hands between contractions and how amazing that was. Finally, after some time, the midwife told me I could bear down if I felt like I needed to during a contraction. I remember this felt awful and good at the same time. AJ reminded me I should move, since I had been on my back in the tub for a while, and we were trying to avoid my cervix swelling like it did with the birth of my second. I tried all fours in the tub, but it was too uncomfortable. I moved to the toilet but didn't have to pee. Instead, my body instinctively started pushing and grunting.

I recognized transition from our classes and I couldn't believe my body was doing exactly what it should. Even in those extremely painful moments, I knew Oliver was coming soon and found amazement that it was all working. Finally, I decided I needed to move to the bed. I tried standing first and then squatting. Nothing was helping. I used the top of the bed as leverage and tried on all fours again on the bed. It was all excruciating. I definitely lost my focus during that time. The contractions were so close together. The pressure was unbelievable. The midwife remarked that my water bag still hadn't broken and that if she broke it, it might help him move down. I remember begging her to break it.

After a moment or two, while still on all fours, the bag broke and warm amniotic fluid poured all over the bed. It was such a moment of relief. I could feel Oliver so close now and asked to lay on my back. I wanted to push. Pushing was incredibly painful. I couldn't seem to feel the correct place to push from and I was in so much pain while doing so that it made it hard to concentrate. I had to remind myself to give in and push despite the pain. At some point the midwife noticed I had a cervical lip. I remember thinking it could be worrisome, just like it was with my second baby's birth. Instead of alerting everyone though, she was able to use her hand and manipulate my cervix to pull the lip away from Oliver's head. It was incredibly painful and it made it very difficult to continue concentrating on pushing.

After 40 minutes of maneuvering the cervix and attempting to push, things were getting close! Everyone was exclaiming that he was right there and that they could see his head. The encouragement helped me gather every bit of strength I had left to continue pushing. The last few pushes just before his head emerged actually brought relief. Suddenly his head emerged and I felt the ring of fire. Although the midwife and nurse remarked afterwards how controlled my pushing had been, I couldn't help but feel the opposite. I remember shrieking and screaming that things were stinging and burning and how painful it really was! After his head was out the last final push was the easiest. His whole body just sort of tumbled out and it was immediate relief.

Instinctively I reached down, felt his little armpits, and pulled his wiggly body right up to my chest. Oliver did not even cry. He had swallowed quite a bit of mucus and was just giving very soft cries. The nurse was able to squeeze out the rest of the fluid from his lungs and nose and airways and he finally let out some pretty hard cries. The midwife responded that I hadn't torn at all and that I had just gotten some grazed abrasions. I was so incredibly happy!

Oliver was taken over to the weigh station and we were told he was born at 2:46am weighing 7 pounds 12 ounces and was 20 inches long! I couldn't believe how tiny he felt even though he was our largest baby out of the three!

I remember feeling very energized immediately after birth and then a few minutes later falling asleep, literally mid conversation with everyone. After what felt like a very long time of skin to skin, we were transferred to another room where we spent time healing and recovering. Overall, it was a fast labor and birth. But the pain was incredibly intense. Despite that, AJ was so helpful, the midwife was incredible, and Oliver was healthy and perfect. I couldn't have asked for a smoother delivery! I was so happy to finally have my baby earthside. Happy Birthday Ollie!

February 21, 2021

Lindsay and Kingston

During pregnancy, my birth plan was to have a home water birth with my midwife. I wanted everything to be as natural as possible and completely unmedicated. I envisioned having a hopefully short labor and delivering my baby boy in water...but Kingston had other plans.

It was a Friday. I was out shopping all day trying to find dresses to fit my bump. I ordered Olive Garden and brought it home for my husband and I. After dinner I started feeling some tightness and cramps. I was only 32 weeks and I had never had Braxton Hicks, so I wasn't sure what the feelings were. The cramps were fairly strong and started coming in waves. I soon realized that I was feeling contractions. On Saturday morning I went to see my midwife to check if my cervix was dilated. She checked and said I wasn't dilated, but my cervix was thinning and was very soft. I continued to have contractions throughout the day and they were all over the place from five minutes apart, down to two minutes apart, up to six minutes apart.

Around 6:00pm my contractions were strong enough that I had to breathe through them. My midwife told me to head to the hospital to get checked out. We got to the hospital around 7:30pm and the OB checked me and I was 2 centimeters dilated. They gave me a steroid shot to help the baby's lungs develop in case I delivered early, and gave me medicine to slow down the contractions.

The medicine to slow contractions didn't work, so they kept me overnight. Sunday morning around 6:00am they checked me again and I was 4 centimeters dilated. At this point it was a waiting game. Because I was in preterm labor, the doctors wouldn't check my cervix again until either my water broke or I felt the urge to push. They just told me to wait and see if the contractions went away or continued.

This was the most challenging part because I had no idea if I was going to have a baby yet or not. I wanted some sort of certainty, but being left in limbo made time pass so slowly and it was agonizing. I was still breathing through the contractions, and around 5:00pm they were coming every two minutes. I asked them to check how dilated I was again, but they wouldn't because they didn't want to do anything that might speed up my labor. They were trying to prolong things so I could get the second steroid injection for Kingston's lungs. At 7:00pm I was in excruciating pain and contractions were one minute apart. I asked what the process was for an epidural.

The nurse told me it could take up to 40 minutes for them to put in the order and for it to take effect. I was in so much pain I didn't think I could make it 40 more minutes. Twenty minutes later I felt the "urge" everyone talks about, and they could see I was in a lot of pain. I'm sure the entire floor could hear me screaming. The nurse came in and checked and I was dilated to 8 centimeters. No one ever talks about "transition," but I can testify it's real. They had to break my water and once that happened, I started to push. This was by far the most painful thing in my ENTIRE life. I was exhausted and thought he would never come. After 20 minutes of pushing, our King was born. He let out the biggest cry and it was the most amazing moment listening to him take his first breath of life.

If I could go back and change things, I wouldn't. The beautiful thing about life is things happen just as they are supposed to. I may have had an idea in my head of what I imagined my birth would be like, but our son came exactly when he was supposed to. He is happy, healthy, and thriving and I am so blessed to call him my son. I also can't thank my husband enough for his endless love and support. We endured the NICU journey together and came out together stronger than before.

February 25, 2021

Sabrina and Lincoln

I was 41 weeks and 5 days. This was the longest I had ever been pregnant, and with the blessing of my midwife, I drank the dreaded induction smoothie. I then quickly got myself to bed hoping for some rest before it started working.

Just after 2:00am I was woken by a strong contraction, and then another. I labored for about an hour before I woke my husband up to let him know I was in labor and things were getting intense quickly. I continued to labor throughout my home before calling my midwife. Due to my history of long labors, I encouraged her to take her time, jump in the shower and do anything else she needed. Then I got in the shower as my husband filled our birth tub. I don't remember much after getting in the shower. Every so often my husband would appear, encouraging me. My sister arrived and supported us. I knew I was in transition when every contraction made me doubt my ability to birth my baby. As my sister reassured me, I looked at her and said, "My perineum is going to fall off." She knew what to do and called my midwife. I moved to the toilet as my body began pushing.

The tub. I had to make it into the tub. I ran in between contractions and my family swears I dove headfirst in, leaving puddles behind me from being soaking wet in the shower. I heard my midwife's voice on the phone, reminding me to breathe through my contractions. So I did. I asked my husband to feel my bottom and sure enough our baby was right there. So very close. At that moment I saw headlights pull into the driveway and that was all I needed to bring my baby earthside. My midwife had arrived and my baby was joining us next!

It felt so good to push. As she walked into our home my sister helped bring birth supplies in and I met her eyes with a guttural growl that every birth worker recognizes from a mile away. As she came to our side she assured my husband, "Great job, if she needs help with shoulders, you can help her." Shoulders?!? I didn't even know our baby's head was born, but there it was in my husband's waiting hands. With one more roar our third son was born from my scarred womb into his father's hands and onto my chest. He quickly announced his arrival with a healthy cry! Our labor lasted just under four hours, despite my preparation for another 36 hour labor. And while my birth supplies sat in the corner, untouched, I was snuggling my fresh baby boy.

My second VBAC baby born at home. Lincoln was 9 pounds 11 ounces. He arrived at 41 weeks and 6 days. Born to Sabrina and Mark.

February 28, 2021

Breanna and Arden: A Birth in New York

In 2018, I was manipulated into an unnecessary induction at 41 weeks pregnant. That induction went poorly and after 3 failed epidurals, a lot of tears, fear, pain, and late decelerations of baby's heart rate, a cesarean was performed. Fast forward to 2021 and I was pregnant with my second son. I knew I needed a different birth experience just as much as I wanted one.

Finding a supportive provider proved to be very difficult; in part because I experienced a complication in my cesarean referred to as Bilateral Uterine Angle Extensions. After interviewing and being denied by multiple providers, I finally found support in the fifth doctor

I met with. It was an obstetrician who runs a stand-alone birth center and practices a midwifery model of care.

My pregnancy went very smoothly. I had a lot of emotional ups and downs. There was a lot to process and work through, but with the help of my therapist, I was confident I was making the right choices for me and my baby. On February 27th I had an OB appointment. I was 41 weeks and 6 days, with no signs of labor starting soon. I requested a pelvic exam and I was a dilated a fingertip, baby was still posterior, and my cervix was very soft. The baby was so low that my OB hilariously noted if he were any lower I would "need a sling just to be walking around." We agreed that we were comfortable waiting until at least 42+6 before considering any interventions.

Later that same day I started having crampy sensations that transformed into mild contractions around 1:30pm. I notified my doula around 5:00 that I thought labor might be starting. I had a good shower, ate a great meal, and decided to get some rest. Sleep came to me around 10:00, but it was short lived. Contractions were getting closer together and more intense. I was waking every ten minutes to ride the waves. Forty-five minutes later I lost my mucus plug. Contractions were localized in my low back, around my hips, and into my groin. At this point I couldn't sleep any more. At 1:40am I woke my partner. I was having a hard time coping alone. My rhythm consisted of vocalizing through contractions while rocking back and forth on my hands and knees with my eyes shut the entire time. We planned to meet my OB at the birth center at 3:00am.

Contractions were intense and every two minutes. I labored all over. On the bed, standing next to the bed, in the bathroom. Mostly on all fours. Lying down was impossibly painful. I tried to labor on the toilet, this intensified contractions beyond belief and also made me feel very pushy – there was so much rectal pressure.

By early morning I was in transition. My doula recommended the birth tub and it provided instant relief. It was exactly what I needed, and I was finally able to rest between the waves. I remember feeling so out of it and so focused at the same time. I was so ready to be done and so proud of how I was coping. My body felt so heavy.

I felt intense pressure and pushed involuntarily at the end of a few contractions. Looking down in the water I saw some bloody show. This made my doula brain very happy and I felt a huge surge of motivation. At 8:00am, with one big push, my waters ruptured! A welcome relief.

After a little while in the tub, I needed a change of scenery. While standing and using ropes hanging from the ceiling as a counterweight, I started to feel lots of stretching and stinging pain. I reached down and felt the squishy, wrinkly top of my baby's head. I started alternating between doing some gentler pulsating pushes and pushing more forcefully. Then his head was born! My body immediately and involuntarily pushed and the rest of him came flying out!

Arden was born at 8:55am. He weighed 8 pounds 15 ounces and was 22 inches long.

A redemptive, unmedicated, VBAC!

March

March 2, 2021

Caylynn and Lyndon

I had had nearly 3 weeks of prodromal labor before my due date with my second baby. I went to the chiropractor, texted with my doula, and tried the Miles Circuit several times. My contractions would last all day and go from every 2-3 minutes apart to suddenly stopping! I was eager to get things moving. I went for a long walk one night and finally woke up on Monday, March 1st with what I knew were real contractions. We had just moved to southern Orange County, but I was still planning on delivering in Long Beach.

I was anxious about a potentially quick delivery since it was my second baby in 15 months, so we decided to drive up to my in-laws' house and labor there for the day. I was in early labor most of the day and did lots of walking around the block and waiting. By 6:00pm I decided I was ready to head to the hospital. We called ahead and checked the visitor policy. Thankfully my husband was allowed to join me in triage.

When we arrived, I was checked in and already 6 centimeters dilated. We were in a room and the nurses thought the baby would come within a few hours since my last labor was pretty quick. But around 8:00pm I "stalled" at 8 centimeters. I was in transition and doubting everything at this point! I had back-to-back contractions that were so painful - way more painful than I remembered with my first. I felt like I couldn't even move or try different positions because I didn't have a break between contractions. I was having really horrible back labor and I constantly felt the urge to push.

At around midnight on March 2nd, I couldn't handle the contractions anymore and made the decision to have an epidural. I went to the bathroom one last time before the anesthesiologist was supposed to come in twenty minutes. The anesthesiologist came in and opened the epidural packaging, I sat up on the side of the bed and felt the baby's head. Before the anesthesiologist could do anything, I yelled, "The baby's THERE!"

My son's head was crowning. They told me I now had to wait for my doctor to come to deliver the baby – which could be another 20 minutes. I told them, "I give a nurse permission to deliver my baby." Turns out there was another doctor that was available down the hall. That doctor ran in and caught my son. He was born at 12:22am within 2 pushes. Turns out he was posterior. I delivered him sunny-side up and that was the cause of a lot of my back labor. I ended up having my second unmedicated birth! Lyndon William Cole, 7 pounds 14 ounces, 20 inches long, born on March 2, 2021, at 12:22am. We are so in love!

March 2, 2021

Danielle and Alexandria: A Birth in Pennsylvania

My daughter ended up making her arrival at 41 weeks and 2 days. I had thought she was going to come sooner. At my 38-week appointment I consented to a cervical check and I was 4 centimeters dilated and around 80% effaced. I definitely did not think I'd be pregnant for three more weeks, but babies decide when they want to come!

The morning of March 2nd I got up and logged on to work. My 2.5-year-old son was already at my mother-in-law's house, so I relaxed and got as much work done as I could while having zero motivation. At this point I was ready for maternity leave. Around 1:00pm I was texting my sister and friends about the obnoxious amount of discharge I was having that day. I even sent a picture of the gray pants I was wearing to show how soaked they were! My sister called me and said, "Do you think that's your water breaking?" and it honestly hadn't crossed my mind.. My water broke first with my son and that was more obvious because it leaked constantly for hours and it had a particular smell. After about thirty minutes I realized it was my water breaking!

I called the hospital around 3:00pm to let them know I was going to come in soon. Normally I wouldn't have rushed to the hospital as early as I did, but since the baby was so low, I really thought she was going to come quick! I got to the hospital around 4:00 and hadn't had any contractions yet. After being triaged I learned I was still 4 centimeters dilated. At that point I regretted going to the hospital so early but tried to make the best of it.

I never wanted an epidural, but it was also never out of the question. Contractions started to pick up a tiny bit but only felt like very mild period cramps. I knew I didn't want Pitocin. I had it with my son's birth and it made my whole labor much more painful. I was very open with my midwives about not wanting it and they were totally supportive. After a few hours of walking around and bouncing on a ball, the midwife on duty came into my room around 8:00pm and asked if I wanted to give the breast pump a try to trigger oxytocin. I said sure!

I knew how to use a pump already, so it was not intimidating, and I figured maybe I could also get some colostrum out. Around 8:30 the nurse brought the pump in. She told me to pump for 15 minutes and then walk around for 30 minutes. Then I should repeat the process and pump on the other side. I finished pumping on my left side around 8:50 and walked around for a few minutes before contractions kicked in. I labored all around the room, but my favorite position was leaning over the bed letting my belly hang parallel to the floor. After about 25 minutes of strong contractions, I was in a lot of pain and had to pee. My husband walked me to the bathroom and while I was in there, I got the urge to poop. Luckily it was really poop and not the baby's head coming out! After that I continued to labor for a few more minutes and called the nurse in. I was in so much pain I wanted to be checked to see if I was progressing. If I wasn't anywhere near being fully dilated, I was considering getting an epidural. I was definitely in transition at this point, and I could physically feel the baby descending through my birth canal.

The midwife came and talked to me about what I wanted to do. I told her I'd like an internal check just to see where things were. At this point I could barely talk and started to sweat. I ended up throwing off my gown and rolled onto the bed. She took a look and said I was 10 centimeters and I could push if I was ready. I had about two to three more contractions and then was holding my surprise baby girl in my arms at 9:35pm. From the time I stopped pumping to holding my baby it only took 45 minutes! I couldn't believe how well the pumping worked and how fast it put me into active labor. It was definitely a great hospital birth experience that I would do again!

Kat and Nathanial

Getting pregnant was never an issue - staying pregnant was. In June 2020, my husband and I sought out a fertility doctor to see why I kept miscarrying. We got no conclusive answers but were told we should do progesterone as a cautionary measure. On June 16, 2020, my egg was ready to release and I ovulated. Three days later I was pregnant and on progesterone. My pregnancy was fairly normal besides the nine weeks of hormones. I did have Hyperemesis Gravidarum and needed IV fluids a few times. I also had anemia and needed iron infusions. I was sent to a high-risk doctor because as a child I had a heart condition. I was medically cleared of my condition when I was 17, but they wanted to be sure there were no problems with pregnancy.

At 38 weeks pregnant my regular OB asked me if I wanted to be induced at 40 weeks and I declined. My plan was a natural birth, no medicine, whenever my baby felt inclined to come. Two days later I had to see the high-risk doctor. He informed me that I NEEDED to be induced because my son would die. I asked why this information was not relayed to me at any of my other weekly appointments. The high-risk doctor also failed to get a second opinion on the issues he said my son had. (My son had and has nothing wrong with him).

After my high-risk appointment I felt angry. I felt like I failed. I called my regular OB to inform them I needed to be induced. They asked me to come in on Monday to schedule the induction, at 39 weeks. I agreed to go and took my husband to the appointment. I waited two hours for them to see me and they came in to tell me that they were informed months ago that I was not permitted to go to 40 weeks pregnant. Again, no one had told me anything. They asked when I wanted to be induced and I suggested Friday. My husband had a 3-day weekend and that gave me enough time to prepare and gave him time to take off the following week. They agreed and went to call the hospital. Then they came back and told me I had to call the next morning at 6 am but probably would not go in until the evening. So instead of waiting until Friday, I was getting induced the next day.

I called the hospital at 6:00am on Tuesday, March 2nd, and was told to arrive by 7:30am for my induction. When I got there, I was informed my doctor was unavailable until 11:30am. At noon he came to see me and started me on Cervidil. I was 75% effaced already but only 2 centimeters dilated. I got another dose of Cervidil at 3:00pm. At 5:00 my husband joined me in the hospital. At 8:00 they told me I was about 4 or 5 centimeters dilated and that they wanted to start Pitocin. I was bouncing on a ball, using a peanut ball and walking around. Overall, I felt pretty good. They kept asking if I wanted an epidural and I said no.

Around this time my hips made an audible crack and I immediately felt funny. I called my nurse who checked and said I was only 5 or 6 centimeters dilated and my water was not broken. By 9:30pm I was contracting hard and fast. The Pitocin was too high and I was fighting my body to not push. The doctor and nurse told me if I pushed at 5 centimeters I would tear my cervix and bleed out. I kept telling them to turn down the Pitocin because I was contracting, but my cervix was not catching up. They finally turned it down and kept pushing me to get an epidural. I declined again.

Around 10:00pm I was ready. My body and cervix were ready and things were in high gear. I felt intense period cramps and the urge to poop. They informed me it was not poop but my son's head. I told them it was a lot of pressure and I wanted to go home. They asked if I wanted medicine. I said some Tylenol in my IV would be fine. The nurse came back and asked if I wanted Stadol, I asked what it was and she said it was basically Tylenol. I had never heard of it and my back was aching, so I agreed.

By 11:30 I was, for lack of better words, high off the MORPHINE they gave me. I was livid that I was given morphine. I was rambling, not making any sense, I kept zoning out. My body does not react well to morphine, and I did not want anything stronger than Tylenol. They said it would help pain not pressure. I kept explaining I was crampy and having and intense pressure in my butt. They said, "Oh, we thought you were in pain."

Anyways, it was too late, and I was loopy, I threw up on my nurse's shoes and was very light headed. Finally, it was time to push. I wanted to watch so the nurse got me a big mirror to see. My husband told me the entire pregnancy he would not look but he did end up watching and recording it for me. I had a ballerina bar across the bed and had my feet up to my chest. I was so uncomfortable and was told I could not stand or move positions. I ended up pulling myself to the bar with a sheet to help get some oomph behind my pushes.

As the ring of fire started, I stopped pushing. I laid back and felt an overwhelming peace. I could feel my body working to help move Nathanial's head. I started apologizing to everyone for being so harsh moments before. My arms were noodles and I could not pull up anymore and I also could not push. I was so tired, but I knew I needed one big push and he would come out. I asked someone to pull the sheet and pull me up. The nurses said it would not help and offered to sit me up from behind. I told them I needed to be pulled, I told my husband to do it and he did. He pulled me up and I told him to pull harder and then out came our son. The nurse said, "Oh maybe she did need to be pulled up."

I was handed our baby and was still a little loopy.

I said, "What is this?"

The nurse replied, "Your baby?"

I said back, "Ugh no it feels like raw chicken and smells weird."

It was our baby, and I was just a little out of it. He was 8 pounds 13 ounces, 21 inches long, born at 1:33am at 39 weeks and 2 days. He was bald as can be and looked just like my grandfather. The birth was not what I imagined. Being loopy and calling my son a raw chicken was not what I had planned. But I am grateful it was fairly quick and painless. There was lots of pressure, but not pain.

March 5, 2021

Kristina and Sayla Sage: A Birth in Florida

On March 5th, at 38 weeks pregnant, I had my first home birth after two hospital births. I had been having prodromal labor for weeks but had some contractions and a little blood that morning. I texted my doula to let her know that it might be the day! I wanted my day to be as normal as possible, so my middle son and I went for a long walk at the park after breakfast. We went home to take a nap and I got woken up by a contraction around 2:00pm. I let Stephen know and told him I wasn't sure if I was in labor or not, but he decided to come home early from work. We ate Chipotle after our nap and around 4:00pm I decided to shower and get all the birth stuff set up just in case.

Around 6:00 we went for another walk, and I had a couple contractions that I needed to stop and breathe through. My friends convinced me to call the midwives and let them know what was going on while I was on my walk. My midwives decided to come check me.

They got to my house around 7:15pm and my midwife checked me and said, "Wait are you sure you're feeling these?"

I said, "I think so. Am I not dilated?!"

She said, "Girl! You're about 7 centimeters!"

I called my doula and continued laboring. Steve and I walked around outside and my amazing doula, Brandy, showed up to save me with some massage. She also let me hold onto her when Stephen wasn't right there. Around 9:30pm it was suggested that I try the birth pool and some pushing. Eventually I got out of the pool because it wasn't comfortable for me at all. I sat on the toilet where I was the most comfortable then moved to the bed. I had always envisioned birthing her in our bed. At 11:17pm Sayla was born. The contractions seemed like a breeze. When she was emerging earth side, I swear my soul left my body to get her here. My whole birth team was amazing and my birth was perfect.

March 7, 2021

Brittany: A Birth in California

I was five days past my due date and had been 4 centimeters dilated for over a week. I woke up the morning of March 7th around 8:30am and felt a contraction. Thy continued and I started to time them. I went downstairs and made a huge breakfast for my family while timing my contractions. They were really irregular and 7-12 minutes apart, but I knew we'd be heading to the hospital that day. I decided to go upstairs, shower, and throw my last-minute items in my hospital bag. While I was blow drying my hair the contractions started getting stronger and I was having to pause and breathe through them a little more. At around 11:00am I began feeling pressure, so I called my doctor and said that we'd be coming in. My husband packed, showered, and we said goodbye to our two older kiddos and my mom. We left at 11:30 and started our 30-minute drive to the hospital.

When we reached the highway, my contractions started coming fast and furious. They were 2-4 minutes apart and I was so uncomfortable sitting down from the pressure. When we got onto the exit ramp, I told my husband I needed to push just to relieve the pressure. His face was one of shock and panic! I pushed a couple of times and felt so much relief. It then hit me that I was in transition and baby was coming FAST. We finally pulled up to the hospital valet, and I practically jumped out of the car, leaving my husband in front of the hospital.

When I walked onto the labor and delivery floor, I was greeted by a nurse. I said, "Hi, this is my third baby, and I feel like I need to poop so we all know what that means!" Every nurse in that quiet hallway turned to look at me. I was taken to a triage room, set my purse down, and immediately went to the toilet. It felt so good to be in that position and after bearing down a couple of times, just as my husband walked into the room, my water broke! I felt my baby come down and I said, "Uh oh!"

The nurse came running in, checked me, and said, "Oh! Baby's right there, we need to get you on the bed!" Before I knew it there were three nurses and the on-call ER OB in my room. I got on the bed and started to push. The only bad part of my experience was when I began feeling some panic from all the staff in the room. It took me out of my zone and into more of a fight or flight state. They didn't even know my name or anything about my pregnancy. I pushed a few times and the doctor asked to perform an episiotomy. I said no and then eventually agreed. Our baby boy was born, adorable and healthy. And with a true knot in his cord! The total time from my first contraction until delivery was only four hours. Our baby was born twenty minutes after arriving at the hospital! We couldn't believe it happened so fast. I was planning a natural birth, and I got it whether I wanted to or not. I am so proud of myself!

March 11, 2021

Abby and Emmett

At 1:30am on March 11th, when I was 35 weeks and 5 days pregnant, I woke up with what I thought were stomach cramps from indigestion. I never expected to have my baby so early and we totally were not ready. We were planning a homebirth and our midwives would not deliver at home before 36 weeks. So, when I had these "cramps", I wasn't thinking about labor. I thought maybe it was Braxton Hicks. I remembered hearing that Braxton Hicks contractions can sometimes be caused by dehydration, so I got up, went to the bathroom, drank tons of water, and laid back down. When I laid back down I noticed that the "cramps" were coming and going at a pretty consistent pace. It was then that I had the first thought that I might be in labor.

At 2:00am I woke my husband up and told him I might be in labor. He asked me if I thought it was food poisoning or if I was overthinking things because I was excited for the baby to get here. He took over timing the contractions and for half an hour we tracked them. When I would lay down, they would come more regularly and consistently with a clear beginning and end. When I would stand up, they seemed to have less clear beginning and ends and seemed to blend together more with the peaks coming further apart.

At 2:15 we called the midwife and were on the phone for twelve minutes. I told her I thought I was in labor and I had been having contractions pretty regularly since 1:30. I had two on the phone with her and when they came, I stopped talking and I breathed through them. After the second one, she told me she was on her way. She said if I was in labor, we would have to go to the hospital because it was too early for him to be born at home. She told us to go ahead and pack a hospital bag. We started packing things in between contractions and it was a little chaotic. While waiting for Jesse to get here, I threw up all the water I had drank. Also, while throwing up, I lost control of my bladder and peed myself. At this point I started to realize I might actually be in active labor because I knew nausea can be common in labor. I took a quick shower when I was finished just to rinse off all the pee and throw up. Then I got dressed and laid on the bed for the next few contractions.

The midwife arrived at 3:11 and called me to let me know she was here. My husband went to let her in. When she came in, I was laying on the bed and she asked to check my cervix. I told her to go ahead and after she checked, she looked up at me and said, "So, you are in active labor. You are six centimeters dilated which is great. You are going to meet your son tonight. Because you aren't 36 weeks yet, the safest thing to do would be to go to the hospital. Your baby is going to be fine, but babies born this early sometimes have breathing difficulties and we want to be at the hospital just in case." I started crying and told the midwife, "We can't have him at the hospital. We're supposed to have him at home. It's too early for him to come." The midwife told me, "I know this is a lot, but he is going to be okay. We should probably get ready to go." I stood up, she listened to Emmett's heart rate really quick, and everything was fine, so I continued to pack.

My husband gave the midwife the car keys and she and I started walking to the car while my husband locked the door and carried the bag. We got to the car and she helped me get into the passenger seat. She said, "If you feel the need to start pushing before we get there, tell your husband to pull over and I'll come help." She followed us in her car and we started driving to the hospital. On the way there, the midwife called them and told them we were coming. She then called my husband and told him to take me to the emergency entrance.

We pulled up to the emergency entrance at 3:41am. On the first floor there was a woman who asked my name, date of birth and some other basic information. By this time, the contractions were so intense, all I could do was close my eyes and breathe or scream through them. I started feeling the urge to push and I told the woman so. A nurse came and wheeled me into the elevator and upstairs to a large room with curtains blocking off individual beds. I took my pants and underwear off and a nurse helped me get onto the bed. Another nurse checked my cervix. After seeing how dilated I was, they did a quick ultrasound to check that Emmett was okay. At some point while in this room, I remember getting incredibly hot and ripping off the sweatshirt I was wearing. The ultrasound looked good and then they wheeled me on the bed into a labor and delivery room.

By the time we got into the labor and delivery room, the midwife was there and I was feeling a very strong urge to push. My husband and midwife were on my left side and the nurse was on my right. The nurse leaned down and said, "My name is Heather and I'm your nurse. Because your baby is so early, there's going to be a lot of people in the room. We have NICU doctors and nurses here and a labor and delivery team here. I understand that you were planning a homebirth and that this isn't what you imagined but it's going to be okay." I looked around and there were a lot of people there. Twelve altogether.

Me, my husband, the midwife, the OBGYN, three OB nurses, a NICU doctor, three NICU nurses.

I started pushing. The nurse kept giving me instructions about how to push but I was too focused on my contractions to really listen to anything she was saying. I just did what my body told me to do. I started pushing with every contraction and soon I could feel that his head was close to coming out. My husband kept asking if he was crowing. The midwife told me when she could see his head and she told me he had hair, I asked what color it was and they said it was wet so you couldn't really tell. I kept pushing and the nurse said, "One more big push and he'll be here." I pushed and Emmet was born!

I remember looking up and seeing the nurse holding him and being in absolute disbelief that this was my baby. That this was the person who had been inside me all those months. He cried right away and they put him on my chest. I had to push a little more to get out the placenta, but it felt like it came out right away. They asked me if I wanted delayed cord clamping and I said yes. They put him on my chest and dried him off and I looked at my son's face. He was born at 4:05am, just over 2 hours after my first contraction, and with only ten minutes of pushing. No medicine or drugs needed. My birth experience was awesome and I hope to do it again someday. It was so fast and intense, but I wouldn't have had it any other day. It made me so proud to be a woman and proud of what my body can do.

March 11, 2021

Dorothy and Heidi

Three days past my due date I woke up with contractions. I've always had a day or so of irregular contractions before active labor begins, so I ignored them and went about my day. They diminished in frequency as the day went on, but I knew my baby would be here soon! I slept well that night until about 2:00am, when contractions woke me. They came every 10 to 15 minutes for the rest of the night. I continued to sleep as much as much as I could in between them. By early morning, I needed to get out of bed and sit on my exercise ball during them. Meg, my 4-year-old, got up around 7:30 and I told her today was the day we'd meet our new baby. She ran upstairs to wake her sisters and tell them. Their enthusiasm was so sweet.

Around 8:00am, contractions started coming every 5 to 6 minutes. Noah was out in the shop, but I wanted someone to be here to help care for the girls and offer moral support for me. I had my mom come as well as a friend from church, Lydia, who was interested in midwifery and excited for the opportunity to attend her first birth. Noah was in and out, checking on me and trying to get things wrapped up in the shop. My mom and Lydia read to the girls and took care of them. They also did counterpressure on my back as contractions got stronger. I always sing during contractions. It helps me stay relaxed and gives me something to focus on. My mom, my daughters, and Lydia would sing along with me some of the time - it was really special.

Noah finally came in the house around 11:00am and I think I was just waiting for him to be with me for active labor to begin. Contractions immediately got stronger and closer together. I was sitting on the bathroom floor in Noah's arms, trying not to throw up like I always do, when I decided we should have the midwives come. I threw up, which I absolutely despise doing, but it gave me confirmation that this was definitely active labor. I got into the tub. I loved the warm water during labor.

The midwives arrived around noon, and things shifted again into even more intense labor (with three more puking episodes). Over the next hour, my hymn singing shifted to loud and frantic praying for strength.

Around 1:00pm I started to feel that icky cervix pinch that I've always had and that I had fervently hoped to avoid this time around. I checked to see and felt baby's head, and, yes, that darn lip of cervix getting squished between baby's head and my pubic bone. I was determined to just breathe through this time and not end up getting a lip held while I pushed again. I tried that for 20 to 30 minutes, but the pinched cervix pain was excruciating, even with not pushing at all. Every time I checked it felt exactly the same. I shifted positions and did all the things without making any headway whatsoever. I felt so out of control with the pain during contractions and like I couldn't possibly handle it anymore. A couple of my poor girls were in tears with the intensity of it and I felt really bad for them and grateful that my mom and Lydia were able to be there with them. Noah was amazing support for me during this crazy intensity, being right next to me so I could hang onto him and he could remind me that yes, I could do this and I was doing well.

Finally, I asked Jen to hold the lip of cervix because I needed so badly to be done with that pinched pain as soon as possible. It was only a handful of contractions with me pushing as Jen held my cervix and the lip was gone. Then my water broke! I was complete at 1:30 and able to just push baby down. I loved this part. It was intense, but I could feel the progress and it felt so good to be getting closer. I remembered how easy pushing and crowning was with my last birth and was happy to have the hard part of labor and birth behind me.

Baby moved steadily down, making progress with every push. I asked Jen for more support on my tissues as her head started to come. I kept my hands on my baby's head to ease it gently out, listening to my body's cues to breathe and allow time to stretch. I didn't feel afraid of that stretching feeling, being pretty confident in not tearing since I never had before. My girls were all crowded in the bathroom with us, and it was exciting for them to get to see baby's head. Her head was born easily. I pushed for the shoulders and said, "I knew it was a good sized baby!" as she was born.

I brought her up to my chest and she cried and I cried and all four big sisters crowded around and just cried and cried for joy. What a blessing to have our sweet baby here! We oohed and aahed over our baby for a few minutes before I asked if it looked like a boy face or a girl face. Meg wanted to be the one to check, so I turned the baby over and we saw that we had another GIRL! Baby Heidi nursed within 15 minutes and we snuggled in the warm tub together and soaked up the sweet brand newness. I called family members while we sat there and nursed. After she was done nursing, Noah held her while I got out of the tub and took a quick shower and enjoyed my quiet minutes alone to be thankful for the safe and wonderful birth of our baby girl.

Then I got to crawl into my comfy bed, where big sisters had laid out their precious handmade gifts of a beautiful baby quilt and knitted hat for their new baby. I ate my usual post birth meal of a breakfast burrito and grape juice. Baby Heidi was weighed and checked over while I ate and family members filtered in to see her.

I loved that she was born in the daytime and all of our immediate family who lived locally could come over in the first few hours for a quick peek at the baby. There's nothing quite so amazing and miraculous as a tiny newborn.

Camilla and Luna: A Breech Birth in Venezuela

An old Venezuelan wives' tale explains how to plan the gender of your baby by observing the moon phases. My first born was a baby boy. In the second pregnancy I desired to have a girl, and planned the exact day of the crescent moon to conceive, and got lucky. I was waiting a little girl. Throughout the pregnancy I felt good (all though I felt pretty weak in between week 6 - 12, which I didn't feel in my first pregnancy). Afterwards I felt active and everything went perfectly well until we turned 34 weeks where our doctor told us that our baby girl was lying very comfortable with her head under my ribs and her back against my cervix. She was laying transverse across me and her head was not down. He told us to wait some weeks to see if she changed her position, which she didn't. We got to week 38 and our little baby still hadn't turned. I am an advocate of natural childbirth and had actually planned a homebirth this time, but the doctors were planning my C-section

We decided to try to turn her into a head-down position, but it didn't work. We did manage to get her out of her position under my ribs and into a full breech position. From then on, I got into a very stressed period of my pregnancy. I got filled with doubt because of all the fear the doctors transmitted. On my own, I started to study about my options to give birth naturally and changed my doctor - but my new doctor also wanted to plan a C-section and told me not to move at all the last two weeks. I got very scared, sad and had a lot of split-feelings. I decided to give it one last chance with a third doctor, who got to be my guardian angel in my birth story. It turned out that she had a lot of experience with breech babies and was willing to help me through a breech birth. Her only recommendation was to give birth in a hospital instead of at home.

At 39 weeks, I felt confident and convinced that I could do it and started again to practice my breath work, visualizations, and relaxation techniques that I knew would be necessary to help in my labor. At 39 weeks and 6 days, at 2:00pm, I felt my first weak contraction. I decided to get the last things ready and at 7:00 I drove my son to my sister-in-law's house. That way I had all night to focus on my contractions. I choose to stay as long as possible at home. I got in to my pyjamas and went to bed to get some rest and my husband did the same. At 11:00pm my contractions started to get stronger and more frequent. I used my breathing techniques and tried to relax my body through every contraction. I also used the verbalization of sounds throughout the pains and meditation, which helped a lot.

At 12:30am I started to feel that I had to get going. We went directly to the clinic where they were waiting for us. My doctor put on relaxing music and gave me a massage to ease the lower back pain. She helped me to remain calm. She couldn't believe that I was already dilated 9 centimeters. That was the only moment she measured. When I started to feel amniotic fluid between my thighs, we got into the operating room where I sat on the stretcher. In that moment my water broke. I felt a strong need to push, so I lifted my legs against my chest in a sideways position.

I felt so much pain. I would say it hurt twice as much as my first birth which was a head-down baby. I tried to stay calm, but I couldn't. I had to scream to release my pain. After pushing three times, the bottom and the legs came out and the pain decreased. Now it was only the shoulders and the head that needed to get out. I felt I couldn't keep my legs open and wanted to shut them, but my husband hugged me and said a prayer into my ear. He grabbed my leg and got it against my chest. In one push, one endless pain, one long and last scream, I felt my baby girl had finally arrived. I saw her and held her. I could finally take a long and deep breath. I felt powerful and proud to stay true to myself and have my breech baby naturally. She arrived at 3:33am and was named Luna (moon). It was a magnificent and unforgettable moment.

March 18, 2021

Mandi and Charles: A Birth in Michigan

Charles George was born at home on March 18th at 4:17am. I was 41 weeks pregnant on Tuesday and we reluctantly made an appointment with our midwives - overdue appointments are never fun. We got dinner first, had our appointment, and Barb reminded us that, "No one is pregnant forever." My Mother-in-law had offered to keep Harper overnight, so Logan and I had a nice little date night. I started having some contractions that felt more real around 9:00pm. I had one every 20 minutes or so and I slept on and off between them from 11:30 until about 4:00am. I got out of bed because contractions were about 6-7 minutes apart and definitely getting stronger. They stayed consistent for several hours and I was hesitant to call Dorothy (my sister) because she had just had her own baby a week earlier. Logan got pretty antsy and said he didn't want to deliver this baby alone, so I called her and she and mom both came around 7:00am.

My contractions stayed the same for a couple hours and then spaced out. I took a shower and a nap and by noon they were anywhere from 8-20 minutes apart again. Logan and I took a walk around the property, and I didn't have a single contraction so Dot and Mom both left. I took another nap and my contractions were still strong but very irregular. I was super discouraged and couldn't seem to stop crying. I took a bath and tried to watch funny videos to take my mind off of my contractions. We attempted to go to bed around 9:00. I hopped out of bed to lean against the wall or the dresser every 15 minutes because my contractions were so intense.

Around 11:00pm my contractions were getting closer so I started timing them again. They were intense and painful and when I hurt, I want my mom, so I called her and said I needed her. Dot came back at 12:15am and my midwife, Barb, arrived at 12:30. At this point the contractions were very intense and the tub had been refilled and warmed up so I got in. For the next hour I rode the waves every couple of minutes and changed positions a lot, trying to get some relief. Leaning on the side of the tub on my knees helped a little because Logan could push on my back and I could hold my mom's hands and yell incoherently in her ear.

Around 2:00am I felt very nauseated after each contraction but never threw up, thankfully. Dot checked my cervix because I really wanted to push but didn't want to make my cervix swell like last time by pushing too soon. I was 9 centimeters dilated, so I breathed through contractions for around 45 minutes. Around 3:30, Dot asked if I wanted to be checked again and I yelled, "YES! PLEASE!" She said my cervix was almost complete and that if she could hold it while I pushed, I could likely get this baby out soon.

So she held it, I pushed, I cried, I said, "Ithurtssobad" and Dot told me to push past the pain, and that it was baby's head moving down. At 3:56 my cervix was back and his head was low! I felt his head and remember looking up in shock because I couldn't believe how fast it was going compared to my first birth. Dot said, "You're not going to push for 7 hours this time!" I looked at Logan and proceeded to sob the exact same words to him. Lots of head was showing and I was blowing and blowing so I wouldn't tear and listening to my body's cues. At 4:12 his head was born and he rotated. At 4:15 I pushed hard but still no shoulders. Dot told me to move to my hands and knees to help baby out, so I not so gracefully changed positions. At 4:17 baby was born! So much relief and so much rejoicing that labor was over!

And then he didn't cry. No noise.

My heart fell into my stomach as I heard them ask my mom for a cookie sheet (to resuscitate him on) and Dot told her to call 911 because our baby boy wasn't breathing. Within 30 seconds, Patrice had begun PPV on him. It was longest 15 minutes of my life. I watched three incredible angels (my midwives and my sister) breathe for my baby, rub him, check his heart tones, and remain so calm. In the background, I heard my mom on the phone with the 911 dispatcher. I was in shock, not even able to cry as I looked at him and touched him and cried out for our sweet baby to take a breath. Dot told me to talk to him, so I started calling him by his name, our boy, our Charlie. Please Charlie, take a breath.

At some point Logan jumped in the tub with me to help hold the cookie sheet with his tiny body on it, so that they could all work as efficiently as possible. After a few minutes he took a few gasps, and we continued to talk to him. At 4:26, they said he was getting a little pinker and added O2 to the PPV. At 4:28 he was taking quiet breaths and his oxygen saturation was 85%.

At 4:30 he was in my arms. At the same time, the first deputy arrived followed by EMS at 4:32. They saw that the incredible birth team had it under control and stayed in the background in case they needed anything.

At 4:36 his lungs were clearing and his oxygen level was 96%.

My dad had woken up around 4, said a prayer for me, and then heard the 911 call on his scanner for a baby not breathing at our address. He tried to call my mom and couldn't get ahold of her and came (flew!) to our house right away. He got there shortly after EMS and I cried when I saw him walk in and see that our baby was okay.

I was clutching Charlie to my chest and felt like I was in a haze. I couldn't stop shaking thanks to the shock and the cold water. At 4:40 I delivered the placenta and was finally able to get out of the now freezing cold tub and into a chair.

I looked at Logan and said, "We have a son!"

I looked around my house at Patrice, Barb, Dorothy, my mom holding my week-old niece, my dad, two EMTs, two deputies - and felt so incredibly thankful for these people who rallied around us. Who all felt relief when Charlie cried for the first time.

Not knowing whether your baby is going to live or die in the next few minutes is a feeling no one can prepare you for. A feeling that I am still processing daily. We are so thankful for the incredible, professional, knowledgeable team at Full Circle Midwifery. They immediately knew what was wrong and took control of the situation. We will forever be grateful to them.

We are thankful for the deputies and EMS personnel and their awesome response time, for their willingness to let the birth team do their jobs, and so thankful we didn't need transport.

March 21, 2021

Bambi and LeRoy

LeRoy was born after a lengthy 28 hours of labor at home, assisted by two midwives and witnessed by my husband. As my first child, I can easily say that both my husband and I had spent the last 40 weeks discussing and planning this exact moment and how we would welcome our child into the world with love and peace in the comfort of our own home. We had known the moment we found out that we were expecting that we would be having a home birth, and that we would wait until delivery to find out the sex of our sweet present.

For two days prior, I was having some prodromal contractions and mild waves of nausea. I had emailed work to let them know that I was out for the count and that I was pretty sure the next time I reached out it would be with baby pictures. I decided to get my mind ready and to turn off outside distractions. I would go through my affirmations with every pressure wave, knowing that these weren't quite what I was supposed to be feeling, but also trusting my body and baby that there was a reason for them.

Saturday morning at 4:00am I felt an honest to goodness contraction. I couldn't say how I knew it was different - I just knew. I started timing them and they were about 15 minutes apart. I went back to sleep after an hour of timing them and woke up at 8:00 to a slightly stronger one. I timed them for another hour and took a screenshot of the timer. I sent that to my midwife to let her know I thought that it was going to be baby day. She called me and reprimanded me for texting her instead of calling her with the big news. I stated that at 15 minutes apart, I thought we had some time to kill.

Around 5:00pm the contractions were around 7 minutes apart and I had already puked twice. I couldn't keep any food down and barely water. We called the midwife with an update and she said that she would be there at nightfall because she was positive we were having a nighttime baby. She walked through the door at 9:00, at the same exact time I had my first 2-minute-long pressure wave. She got some water in me and sent me to bed while she and my husband turned our living room into my dream birthing room.

My husband hung up twinkle lights and posted affirmations all around the living room while my midwife filled up the pool, laid down the towels and got her tools ready. At about midnight I woke up to my body ready to go. I had three very strong waves just 2 minutes apart and my body didn't want to lay down anymore. I started walking the hallway and around the living room. After a couple laps at about 1:30am we decided to get me in the pool to see if the water would help things progress. It didn't. I was having so much pressure that it hurt to sit on my butt. I still wasn't fully dilated and my sac was blocking the canal. My midwife decided to break my waters so we could get some progress, and shortly after I said the thing that she had been waiting for - "I have to use the bathroom." I went to the toilet and labored on it, trying to hide the fact that I was pushing. My husband was attempting to counter pressure my back and he kept telling me not to push on the toilet. My midwife caught on and pulled me off to check. I was still not stationed. She let me labor naturally for another hour but I was so dehydrated and exhausted from puking everything up that she decided to step in.

I was laying on the couch with the peanut ball between my legs thinking to myself that I just couldn't do it anymore. I was so tired, my entire body ached, and it was trying to expel my child but nothing was happening. I thought that I just didn't have the ability. I remember weakly repeating "I don't want to do this anymore." Suddenly my body felt different. I looked around and could see me, on the couch looking at me. I was so pale and tired.

Then I heard several voices saying, "You can do this, you got this." Then all of a sudden, I was back in my body on the floor, my midwife telling me that we were going to have to get physical to get this baby out and that I needed to give more strength to this than anything else I've ever done in my life. My baby was stuck. I was on my back, one leg on one midwife, one leg on the other and my husband behind me. I was curling my back with every wave to help push the baby down.

My midwife had to reach up and manually rotate my child over my tailbone and under my pelvis in a corkscrew motion to unstick the head and shoulders. Baby came out fast and easily after the shoulders were unstuck. He had been in the vaginal canal too long and had swallowed some meconium. He didn't cry right away. I called out as soon as he was born, "I knew he was a boy!" I had known the whole pregnancy that it was a boy based off a dream I had at 9 weeks. My midwife cleared his throat and nose and gave him a quick rub and a cry came out as he was put to my chest. He crawled up and immediately started nursing while my midwives prepared for the placenta.

Unfortunately, that is where everything went wrong. My midwife pushed down on my tummy and told me I was going to have to push just as hard as I had been a few more times. I tried. Twice I bore down- and nothing happened. She gave a gentle tug and the entire cord broke away from my placenta. I was given two shots of Pitocin to see if that could help staunch the bleeding and help get the placenta loose. The second midwife called emergency services for a retained placenta and possible hemorrhaging. We were told 10 minutes and all I could think was "At least I am getting 10 more minutes with my beautiful son."

When EMS showed up about 6 minutes later I was still naked. The firefighters were first on scene and came into the house to warn us that it had snowed and the gurney couldn't make it to the door. They asked if I could walk or if I would need to be carried. I stated I could walk just fine. My husband grabbed me an old shirt and his robe and helped me put them on. Then I was walking off to the ambulance, leaving my newborn with my husband. After being asked several questions to verify my mental stability, I was being whisked to the hospital.

I was given an epidural and joked with the anesthesiologist about how after what I just went through- a giant needle in my back was nothing. The D and C showed my placenta had ruptured and was breaking off in little pieces. I asked the doctor that since I was numb and she was already down there if she could stitch me up since I just had a big baby boy - she said there wasn't enough of a tear to warrant a stitch.

When I was out of the OR and back in my room, my midwife was there waiting for me. She was able to take the reins and called my husband and made sure I was fine. It was then she told me that I had pushed out a 9 pound, 12 ounce boy with a 15 inch head and 21 inches long and that he was on his way to the hospital to be with me. It definitely didn't end the way I had planned, and in the end I still ended up knowing how miserable Pitocin and an epidural are. But my boy came earthside at home, healthy as can be, and that was worth everything.

March 22, 2021

Esmeralda and Emerie: A Birth in Illinois

At 1:00am I lost my mucus plug. I began feeling sporadic surges around 4:00. By 7:00 I noticed they were not going away, so I started timing them. They continued throughout the day but were very inconsistent and anywhere from 5-20 minutes apart. On average it was about 10 minutes. I was in complete denial that this was real labor because of the inconsistency. However, the surges were getting stronger and longer. I had been texting my mom and doula all day to keep them updated just in case contractions picked up. Around 4:30pm I finally believed that this wasn't going to stop, so I called my aunt who would be watching my son when it was needed.

Everyone got to my house around 5:00pm and I texted my doula to head on over at 5:30 because I could no longer talk through my surges. When she arrived, we talked for a bit and then headed upstairs to my birthing space. Surges started to get very close together at this time, so we decided to start filling the tub since I wanted a home water birth. Around 6:45 I had my husband help me up from the floor to the bed because the pressure got very intense. I had one surge on the bed and - pop - my waters broke and I could feel her bulging out! I was still wearing clothes so I had to yell for my mom and doula's assistance and I just remember saying, "Take everything off she's coming out!" Sure enough, they pulled off my pants and there was her head. I didn't even have to push because the Fetal Ejection Reflex took over very quickly, not even a minute later, and at 6:50pm Emerie was born.

March 23, 2021

Bria and Hugo

Baby number three was due on March 14th, but my birthing history told me we wouldn't likely meet them before their due date. I planned to go late, so I wasn't disappointed when my due date passed. After a week of prodromal labor, contractions finally started to get serious around 11:00pm on March 22nd and I was able to sleep through them until about 2:00am. At that point I got up and made myself a bowl of oatmeal, but didn't feel like I needed to wake my husband or my birth team yet.

My kids and husband woke up in the morning, and my doula team joined us. The contractions continued slowly and steadily throughout the day. By midafternoon, my midwife suggested I take a nap. I dozed for about an hour (waking every 10-12 minutes for a contraction), and when I got up things really started to progress.

We filled the birth tub around 4:30pm, and expected the baby to join us for dinner. I'm not a quiet birther – I roared through every contraction as my team provided counterpressure to offset the back labor. I could feel myself hitting a limit after a few hours of active labor, so I climbed into the birth tub. Once settled in the tub, I put my hands on my belly and whispered, "Baby, we're taking a break." I had no concept of time, but my team told me the contractions that had been coming every 2-3 minutes ground to a complete stop. After about 15 minutes of rest, contractions came back in full force. Experiencing the mind-body connection, and bond between myself and my baby, was the most powerful part of my labor.

My midwife suspected that the baby was on my right side, and was slowly working themselves into a more optimal birth position. For the next three hours, my team directed me into various positions to help the baby rotate. This part was grueling, and the hardest thing I have ever done. My doula gave me a hair comb to clutch in my fist, which helped distract my mind and allow me to relax my lower half.

At 10:15pm, I yelled at my team that I was done with their moves, nobody was allowed to touch me, and I pushed past them all into my bathroom shower. I sat on an exercise ball in the shower, with hot water pouring onto my back and I lost all mental resolve. My doula peeked her head in and I told her to call the hospital and tell them we were headed in for an epidural. She smiled, knowingly, and I resisted the urge to punch that smile right off her face.

In the next few minutes, my mind left my body completely. When I came to, I was standing up, holding onto the towel bar, and there was a baby on the floor of the tub - amongst blood, amniotic fluid, meconium, and my midwife's hands. Hugo was born in one push at 10:22pm on March 23, 2021.

Just like that, we became a family of five.

March 26, 2021

Madeline and Jude

I knew that Jude was going to be born on time. I told my midwife that I knew he would be here very close to his due date, which was March 27th. She responded with, "Well, no one ever thinks their baby is going to be late, so we will see. Don't be surprised if you end up carrying for another couple weeks. That is very common with first time moms." I thought that was a funny comment because I'm sure it was true, but I still just had a feeling.

On March 25th around 11:00pm, I was laying on the couch with my husband watching Audrey Hepburn in Funny Face when I felt a pop. It was almost like someone had popped a balloon inside me. I could have sworn I heard it out loud, but my husband was only startled by the look on my face. I sat up slowly and he asked me what was wrong. I told him I wasn't sure but that I thought my water just broke. He helped me stand up and sure enough water came trickling out of me and soaked my sweatpants. I went and quickly sat down on the toilet and called my midwife. When we spoke, she asked me to describe what I saw, to which I said a whole bunch of water and small white pieces everywhere. She confirmed that my water had broken and told me to go to bed and get some sleep because the baby was coming either that night or the next day.

There was no chance I was getting any sleep. My contractions started right away and between that and the excitement I couldn't relax or keep my eyes closed. My husband didn't get any sleep either, not from the lack of him trying. Every time I had a contraction, I squeezed his arm and he would wake up. I called my midwife around 1:30am when my contractions started to get stronger. I told her my contractions were 6 minutes apart and were lasting about 1 minute. She told me to give it some more time and I would know when to call her back.

Since we were living with my in-laws, my husband ran a bath for me in their jacuzzi tub right next to our room, as it was deeper than the one in our bathroom. The water felt so nice on my body. The warm water instantly soothed me and made the contractions less intimidating. I stayed there until around 4:00am and then decided to call my midwife back. I told her my contractions were 3 minutes apart and were lasting 1 minute. She coached me through some contractions over the phone and told me to make low 'mooing' noises through each surge. It sounded silly and I'm not sure it really helped, but it gave me something to focus on and I did it from that point onward. I don't think anyone in the house got any sleep that night.

When my midwife showed up, I had been out of the bath and gotten back in again. She had brought an assistant and they both came into the bathroom and checked my blood pressure and the baby's heartbeat. They did this every 30 minutes. Before my labor started, I remembered thinking I would wear a sports bra the whole time as I was very afraid of being naked in front of people. When the time came, that was the last thing on my mind. I didn't even care if I accidentally flashed my husband's family as we were moving from the jacuzzi tub to our room. If they saw me, it didn't matter. I was performing a miracle and couldn't care less.

My husband never left my side. That is one thing I remember vividly. I can only recall him leaving for a few seconds to go to the bathroom or quickly update everyone waiting in the living room, but he was always back before the next contraction. He was by my side or pushing on my hips to try and relieve the pressure. Then all of a sudden, I wouldn't want to be touched and he would just sit there with me. He made sure I drank water and distracted me when I needed it. He told me afterwards that he felt so useless the whole time, but him being there, a person that I completely trusted, was the most incredible support.

I moved to our bed and the midwives had made it up with pads, towels and tablecloths to clean up any mess. I really don't remember lying in bed that much. Labor was such an incredible thing- I was more in the moment than any other time in my entire life. I don't have a high pain tolerance at all. I cry when I get needles or have to get blood drawn. This was so much more intense and yet I knew I could do it. I remember saying out loud, "I can do this," over and over again. Afterwards, people teased me about this as they could hear me all morning saying those words, but it helped so much. In hindsight, I can now see how incredibly important it is to have a strong mind going through labor and I'm proud of myself for never wavering in my confidence. If I had let even the smallest bit of doubt creep in, I can tell you that things might have gone downhill very quickly. I was in this beautiful mental state and I was going to have my baby. That was the outcome that I wanted, so I focused on it.

The midwife asked me if I wanted her to check my cervix and I agreed to let her. She told me I was about 9 centimeters dilated. I was so ecstatic because I thought that meant I was almost there! Wrong. I felt the urge to push and listened to my body and started to. I pushed and pushed but nothing seemed to be happening. She did another cervical exam and found that a little lip of my cervix was still in the way, and I had made it inflamed by pushing on it.

My midwife gave me arnica pills and put ice in a rubber glove and applied it to my cervix and tried to lift it while I pushed in an effort to bring the swelling down. It wasn't working fast enough and she told me I would have to stop pushing while the swelling decreased. Of everything in my whole labor experience, that was the most difficult. Breathing through the overwhelming urge to push with each contraction was almost impossible. I knew I had to do it to bring the swelling down and deliver my baby, but some urges were just too strong and I had to push. My midwife would tell me, "Okay you can try pushing again in 10 more contractions." I would count them down with my husband and she would conveniently slip an extra one or two in there every now and then, which I caught onto right away.

After about 1.5 hours of not pushing, my swelling had finally gone down and I could start pushing again. A new challenge presented itself - I had no idea how to push. I had never pushed something out of that hole before and had no idea what muscles to use. All I was doing was pooping, which my midwife swiftly wiped away. My husband had no idea I had done that until I told him afterwards. My midwife put her fingers inside against my cervix and told me to push her fingers out of me. That really helped as it gave me somewhere to focus my energy. Things started to move along. I must have pushed for about 2-3 hours in total but after the first 30 minutes my husband could see the head and told me he was almost there! I was so excited, until the midwife said, "Well you're doing a really good job, but we still have a ways to go."

With every contraction I gave three big pushes. The midwife and her assistant let me push my feet against their bodies and my husband held my hand. My midwife told me to put my hand on my baby's head and push back to provide counter pressure. This was done to ease his head out slowly so I wouldn't tear. I will admit it felt sort of slimy and creepy to touch at first, but I eventually started to feel the connection of touching my son's head. I could feel my body stretching over him. At first it was disheartening because with every push his head would come out a little but then go back in. Eventually I kept that pressure through the breaks and we made real progress.

When my contractions came every 30 seconds the breaks were just enough to let my body stretch and prepare to relieve the incredible burning sensation that came with every push. Then all at once, the head was out and as my midwife told me to keep pushing his whole body just fell right out of me in a matter of seconds. My husband quickly caught him under his arms and put Jude on my chest. The first thing my baby felt when he started to come out was his dad's touch, not some stranger looking at him under bright lights. Jude was with both of us in our little room, safe in our bed. It was the most incredible feeling in the world and difficult to put into words now. My husband and I cried and laughed, felt relief, exhaustion and elation all at once. I will never forget that feeling. After 13 hours I delivered my 9.3 pound baby boy at 2:34pm on March 26, 2021. Beautiful, healthy, perfect, right on time and within a few hours of his predicted due date.

The mind of a mother is so powerful. Our bodies will do anything we tell them to if we whole-heartedly believe we can. We bring life into this world and I will forever be in awe and so grateful to my mind and body for growing this perfect little person. I've gained such a respect for myself and when I look in the mirror and see all of my imperfections - my floppy arms, saggy belly and sore nipples - I think wow, what a strong, beautiful body! That is the gift my son has given me in return.

April

April 8, 2021

Krista and Odin

Odin was born on April 8, 2021, at 8:48pm. He was born in a birth pool in our bedroom. My due date was April 9th, and I was shocked to make it a day shy of 40 weeks since my first was born at 37 weeks. I started having contractions 5 minutes apart at 35 weeks and so I fully anticipated Odin to come early. He had other plans, and for 5 weeks I had frequent contractions for hours. They would stop for a few hours at night, but I was on high alert. I was gentle on my body and mind and knew that the last weeks can be the hardest mentally. I gave myself lots of grace and reassurance as I waited.

Our room was beautifully set up. We had the birth pool ready, the twinkle lights, candles, favorite pictures, towels, and birth affirmations around the room. Every nap time I would take a picture of my 19-month-old just in case it was the last picture of him as an only child. I was really sad at the idea of him no longer being my baby, and I knew a newborn would make my baby grow up in a way that we couldn't change back. Little did I know how incredibly GOOD that change would be. Orion and Odin are the best of brothers!

At 38 weeks, my contractions were stronger and more frequent to the point I called my aunt and birth photographer to our home. They were there all day but by the evening I knew it wasn't time and sent them home. I was a bit frustrated but also relieved that my support system was gracious and in no rush. They honored me and my space.

Two weeks later on April 8th I was up taking one of my thousand nighttime pees when I noticed a slight trickle was still going even when I was done. I had a hairline leak! That meant my waters were starting the process of breaking and that a baby coming would soon be my reality. This was at 3:00am. I went back to bed, told my husband, and tried falling back to sleep...except I couldn't. It was uncomfortable laying down and I needed to move. So that's what I did! I got up and enjoyed the morning sunlight coming through our windows. Each contraction excited me! Every strengthening and tightening meant that my body was doing exactly what it needed to do. Odin was working with the contractions and feeling him move and work with my body was amazing. We finally got to do this thing and I was excited! My mindset was prepped and ready for labor. This was the homebirth I wanted.

I called my photographer who lived over an hour away and told her she should head over. I called my aunt and told her the same. We had a beautiful, lovely day - eating, chatting, snuggling my toddler, dancing to music, and watching the crazy weather. We had sun, rain, and hail that day and it was perfect. Each contraction had strength and was building slowly with intensity. I looked forward to the next one. I imagined what it was doing, helping open my cervix that was already soft.

Around 6:30pm I had a strong craving for these specific cookies followed by a flood of tears and sobs. I was a puddle of tears crying for these cookies. My husband had me in a big hug and was trying to understand me. I hadn't been emotional like this until this point. I was distraught that I had been stupid enough to eat the whole box a couple weeks back.

"How could I have been so stupid?! I ate the whole box but I want them now!"

So, off my aunt went in search of those cookies…

I calmed down a little bit and knew that someone was going to bring me cookies so I'd be alright. At 7:30pm, in the same spot next to my bed that I had cried over the cookies, there was a huge pop and the rest of my waters broke all over the floor. My husband ran in with towels and held me as I had a huge contraction. We were both laughing and crying the way we did when my waters with Orion had broken! It was so fun! I knew what this meant for me - there's no going back. The thing about a second baby and being a doula is that I knew I was going into transition and that baby was close. I ran to the bathroom to let the rest of the waters continue to come out and pee while I had the chance. My husband and toddler were with me, excited and encouraging! I had the midwife on speaker giving her an update. She asked me if she should come over and I was like oh no, that's okay go ahead and wait... and then I had a heavy contraction followed by a heavier contraction. I moaned, "Yeah actually maybe you should head over." She completely agreed. My aunt made it back to with the cookies, but I was too far into transition to want them or even realize she was back. My toddler though... in every photo of me during transition, he has a cookie in his hand or mouth

The pool was filled and ready, so I hopped in. I wanted to save the warm water for when I needed it the most and this timing was perfect. It was nice to have the weight off my feet. These contractions were far more intense and less spread out. It took focus to go through these ones. I was very loud. My husband was on the outside of the pool holding me and speaking encouraging words to me. He was waiting for me to tell him when to get in, because the plan was for Orion and him to be in the pool while I pushed. My first birth was traumatic and I don't remember transition. This birth I wanted to be different. I wanted to be present and aware of transition. This time around I had midwives that agreed to no cervical checks unless I asked and to be hands off. Transition contractions are next level for me and I relied on my husband to help center me and keep me in the moment. At one point I scratched his back as I held onto him as hard as I could. Between those intense contractions, I would enjoy the calm, the peace, the break - it was my short time to rest.

My midwife asked if I wanted to just feel for myself with my finger what was going on inside. I loved that idea! I put a finger inside thinking I'd feel a head ... nope. Nothing. I couldn't feel him at all. Suddenly a big contraction came on and Odin came full force down on my finger and pushed my finger OUT and his head was emerging! I was in the water on both knees, leaning on the edge of the birth pool with my husband in front of me. I looked over at the midwife and said, "Fetal Ejection reflex! He's coming out!"

He could have come all the way out right there, but I knew to slow down and breathe to give my perineum some time to stretch with him. I breathed, re-centered, put one foot in front of me for balance, and then pushed him out with the strength of the next contraction. He slid beautifully into my hands and I pulled him up with joyful surprise at how amazing that just was. There was no time to get my husband or son in there with me. I went to the other side of the pool to rest on my bottom while I brought Odin up to my breast and he started suckling and licking - discovering his new surroundings. He had dark beautiful eyes with an scrunched up grumpy old man look. Kevin, my husband, brought Orion close and we all experienced the bonding love that comes in that immediate birth high.

Kevin put Orion in the birth pool with me. He had watched birth videos with me multiple times a week leading up to Odin being born. He knew the process of birth and was excited when I was in labor and would point to the birth pool telling me to get in - he knew if I got in a baby would come out.

I felt my contractions pick back up and the placenta was ready to come out. I sat up into a kneeling position and with my right arm holding Odin on my chest I pushed out the placenta and caught it with my left hand. The first push brought it halfway out and so then I just gently pushed and the rest popped out. With Odin on me and a midwife carrying his attached placenta in a bowl, I got out of the pool and into bed. Orion and Kevin snuggled up to Odin and me while Odin nursed. Kevin cut the cord awhile later when it was white and limp. Odin weighed 7 pounds 4 ounces and was 21.5 inches long. He came out 1 hour and 15 minutes after my water had broken. It was a dreamy healing redemptive birth!

April 13, 2021

Kelsie and Baby Girl

We had no idea going to bed Monday night that we'd be waking up to the experience of a lifetime. That night I went to bed with some mild cramping around 11:00pm, but nothing that made me think she would be coming soon. It just felt like some bad period cramps. Layton and I headed to bed while Daddy was working on the flooring trim in our living room. Darren finally came to bed around 1:30am and I told him I was still having cramps. I was able to sleep through them, so I didn't think much of it.

I woke up around 2:50am from the cramps and decided to go pee. When I came back from the bathroom (ours is in remodel so I walked across the driveway to my mother-in-law's house), Darren asked me if he needed to get up and get stuff ready for our home birth. I still didn't realize I was in active labor. I just thought I had really bad cramps going on. Like Braxton Hicks. But he got up and decided he needed to start thinking about getting everything ready. I called our midwife, Naomi, around 2:55am. We talked for about 5 minutes and came to the decision she was going to come over and check me. After we hung up, I called my mom to let her know to stay by her phone.

Next, I woke up Darren's mom before I walked over to him and let him know my midwife was on her way to check me. When I say this man and I make a great team, I mean it. He grabbed my diffuser and put oils in it for me. He was also trying to figure out how we could fill the pool since we hadn't done a "dry run" yet to see how it all set up. I felt like I needed the bathroom again, so I went to the bathroom and Brenda, Darren's mom, was up cleaning a few things. I was really starting to feel the uncomfortable cramping, the real ones. I spent most of my time on the toilet, but did get on all fours at one point. That's when Brenda decided she would go get Darren.

Thankfully she did because our little girl was out in no time after this. When she walked to go get him, I could feel I was about to start pushing. Darren made his way to the bathroom and tried to fill the bathtub so I could still have the water birth I wanted. I told him there was no time.

He bent down in front of me on the toilet to get a better look at how close I was, and he could see her head crowning. In those quick moments my water burst all over him and the floor! Both a little scared, we looked at one another and went into action mode. I had one contraction after my water broke and that got her head out with no problems. Not wanting her to fall in the toilet, I reached down and grabbed her and she came right out into my arms. She was here! Just ten minutes before my midwives arrived. We immediately called the midwife and told her so she could walk us through what to do until she arrived.

My placenta had fallen right out (thank goodness for gravity) into the toilet. Our biggest concern was getting it out of the toilet. I stood up so Darren could reach under me and full handed grab the placenta out of the toilet. We noticed how short her umbilical cord was. We held it in a chucks pad until our midwife arrived and we were able to cut the cord. The first midwife arrived and looked at us from the hallway and had to stop and take a candid photo. In her 13 years she had never had this happen! I feel super blessed that my man and I worked so well as a team to bring our baby girl into this world.

It was nothing like what we had planned or even talked about, but it was beautiful and I wouldn't want to change anything.

April 14, 2021

Valerie and Gary

The contractions started at 40 weeks and 2 days. They varied in frequency from 8 minutes apart to 30 minutes apart. My husband, Blake, referred back to our Bradley Method classes and we did some of the activities they recommended if you thought you might be in early labor: eat something, drink something, take a walk, take a shower, try to nap. Blake wanted me to call the midwife. We agreed that if I had an increase in the intensity, I would let her know what was going on.

Around 6:15pm I had the third really intense contraction. We texted our midwife, Amanda, and she said it sounded like the real thing. She told me to try to get as much rest as I could as it could still be a while and she wanted me to save as much strength as possible. We went to sleep around 11:00pm and I was having more painful contractions every 8-15 minutes as I tried to get some sleep. Around 2:00 I woke up to contractions I could not ignore. I woke my husband up and told him I thought this was it. He immediately jumped in to getting our room ready: putting a waterproof layer under our sheets, putting down tarps, blowing up the birthing tub, and setting up a pot to boil herbs. He even set up candles and put classical piano music on in the background. It was warm and peaceful to labor in our room.

I labored in bed with Blake until around 5:30am. Our midwife got to the house just before 6:00 and suggested I get into the shower on the birthing ball to help me relax. The contractions were more intense, but still spaced 4-5 minutes apart. I started laboring in all different positions: on the toilet, standing next to the bed, holding on to Blake. I finally got into the tub around 8:30am. It was such a welcome relief. I was warm and my contractions slowed down a bit to 8 minutes apart. I ate an apple with almond butter, drank tea and water, and just rested. An hour later the midwife said we needed to get things moving again. We walked up and down the stairs, did some cat/cows, and then landed back on the bed. I started to go through transition around 10:30am. I felt I could not go on during every contraction.

Around 11:30am the contractions were so intense I could not control the urge to bear down and push. I was pushing through contractions, but there was not much progress. My midwife suggested

I use gravity to help. She asked me to move to the toilet again. Once there, my pushing became more effective. I could feel my pelvic floor opening. The baby was not passively being pushed out at this point. Every time I felt a contraction starting, he would push his legs straight up to the top of my uterus as the contraction would squeeze down. He was helping me get him out.

We moved to our final position on the bed. I was kneeling with my upper body on the birthing ball. My doula (who is also my sister) was at my head- holding on to my hands as I pulled on her with all my strength during every contraction. Blake was massaging my back and watching the progress as I pushed. I pushed and pushed until his head started crowning. I could feel him move down through my pelvis and through my soft tissue, but then move back up while I was resting. My birth photographer told me this was what needed to happen. It was allowing my tissue to stretch slowly so I wouldn't tear. I was so done with pushing at this point.

The contractions were lasting long enough for me to push 2 or 3 times with each one. I asked Amanda how many more times I would have to push to get him out. She said, "Less than you've already done." Two contractions and 5 pushes later, he was out to the widest part of his head. At this point I could not hold back anymore and gave one last strong push. At 1:16pm, Gary shot out. It was an indescribable sensation of intensity and immediate relief as he emerged. The rest of his head, body, and amniotic fluid gushed out into Blake's hands. Gary immediately started crying and flushed pink with his first breath. I was in shock that he was here so quickly. I almost couldn't move. My sister helped me get off the ball and onto my back, where they placed Gary on my belly. He was so sweetly crying and clearing his lungs perfectly.

Immediately after giving birth, Gary and I got time to cuddle while we waited for the cord to stop pulsing and my placenta to detach. His newborn exam showed his heart and lungs sounded perfect. He weighed 7 pounds, 2 ounces and was 20.75 inches long.

April 15, 2021

Fransisca and Faeriella: A Birth in France

I knew I wanted a natural birth with my first baby - as natural as possible with no epidural. I found out about water birth, but it's not common in France. I found one maternity hospital that has a birth tub in their service and it's around 1-2 hours by car from where I live. I gave birth to my first baby there, but I couldn't use the birth tub because somebody else was already in that room. I was so upset. It was a long labour. The midwife broke my water and put me in the standard position on the table. Our baby had difficulty coming out and they called the doctor and talked about forceps and caesarean. I started to have doubts, because I was so tired. My husband still believed in me, and he said loudly while holding my hand, "I trust you. You can do this." After I heard that, I felt my cervix open like flowers blooming and with one wave, my baby came out before the doctor even got to the room. I was so glad and relieved.

For my second baby I read more books about birth. I knew I wanted to have a home birth and my husband preferred with a midwife. In France there are only a few midwives that will assist with home birth, and it's not covered by mutual or assurance (so it will be so expensive!). We struggled to find a midwife. While searching I found a Facebook group about home birth and kept reading lots of birthing books. I gained confidence in my body and about birth and decided I didn't want someone else to tell me how to birth. I listened to my instincts, did yoga, and said mantras every day. I ate healthy and decided to have an unassisted birth.

It was 7:00am when I woke up in the arms of your papa. I felt I wanted to take a nice warm bath and eat watermelon, so I told him so. He asked me if this is the time? I responded, "Don't ask me, I don't want to wake up my neocortex with reflection to answer that question." It started gently. Your big sister woke up and joined us eating watermelon in the bathtub. Labor got stronger and stronger. Every time the water became cold, I went to the bedroom and I hung on to your papa. When he was not there, I would hang on the bed sheet. Sometimes papa offered something to eat and drink. Sometimes your big sister made me laugh and we made a choir of AAAaaaaaaaa to open my mouth. I also shared some deep kisses with your papa when your sister went out to play (mouth open = cervix open).

My water broke in the bathtub. I was really amazed how it broke because it was like a bomb in the water. After that it was really fast. I went to go poop and after that I felt your head come out. I held your head while putting my other hand and feet on the floor like a yoga position cat-cow. Papa came and held your head while I waited for the next wave. With just one more wave you came out! The warm hands of Papa welcomed you to this world and then he put you to me. I hugged you tightly and said, "Oh my baby, we did it, yes, you are here with us in this world now, with Mama, Papa and Cici Gigi!" And then you responded to me and you cried! Papa cried too.

After we were sure you were okay, we went to the bedroom beside the bathroom and put you to my breasts where you instantly started nursing. Around 5-10 minutes after you came out the placenta came out. We let you decide when you were ready to say goodbye and let go of the placenta and did a lotus birth. Everything was wonderful.

I didn't bother to know what time you were born nor your measurements or your weight. You were born gently around 2:00pm in our bathroom. Your big sister and Papa are the witnesses. It was so beautiful outside that the cherry tree in the garden was beautiful in bloom to welcome you in with the beauty of spring. Oh my little Fae, you bring us magic in our life from your birth.

April 16, 2021

Kara and Jasper

It was the morning of April 15th and 5 days past my "due" date. I was outside enjoying the warmth of the morning sun, watching my 2-year-old play in the dirt while I crossed off the last things on my "to-do" list before baby would arrive. It happened to be refreshing myself with "Ina May's Guide to Natural Childbirth."

I had been experiencing Braxton Hicks for the last two days, praying they would start to wrap my body and turn into a real contraction. "Breathe, release, surrender." I rehearsed affirmations in my head. "Trust your body, trust your baby, all in divine timing. All in divine timing." As I walked inside to fix lunch, I felt the first contraction wrap. It was 11:00am. I was instantly excited. "Take it slow, trust that they will continue to wrap. Trust that this is it." I told myself as I prepared for the work ahead. As the day progressed and my contractions continued consistently, I called my husband to let him know I was in the early stages of labor, at home, with our son.

I ate lunch and continued to keep myself moving, cleaning, and doing. I wanted these to stay consistent. Around 3:00pm my husband arrived home from work. My contractions were consistent, but not intense yet. I walked the yard barefoot, welcoming each wave. As the night fell, I tucked my son into bed. With a good-night kiss, we told him he may wake with us gone to have the baby.

I worked tirelessly through the night. Swaying and breathing through each wave. As the early morning hours approached and the intensity increased, so did the exhaustion from little to no rest throughout the night. It was almost 6:00am and it still wasn't time to leave for the hospital. My son would soon awake to find me in the tub working through each intense rush as they came closer and closer together. We excitedly explained that the baby would arrive soon. As my son fed me toast in the tub, I sobbed knowing this would be our last moment as a family of three.

At 7:30am on April 16th my bloody show appeared as I sat on the toilet to help my body further dilate. My contractions were now less than 5 minutes apart. It was time to call my sister so we could leave for the hospital. We arrived at the hospital at 9:00 and as I stepped out of the vehicle, I felt a gush! My water had started to break! By 9:30 a triage nurse had hooked up monitors. She also checked my cervix with permission. I was 7.5 centimeters dilated and 100% effaced. My midwife was called and she said she was about 10 minutes away.

At 10:30 it was time to get into a delivery room. My contractions were 3 minutes apart and growing into transition intensity. My nurse watched as my husband and I worked through each wave together, swaying, and moving baby down with each moan. I asked for my midwife and nurse to give us some time to work through these next few alone. I knew I had some time.

By 11:00am I was working through contractions, moving back and forth from the toilet to the bed. I was lunging through each contraction to get my birth canal open to bring baby earthside. My midwife had me on my side laying in the bed with my knee up on a peanut ball to open the pelvis. After 2 transition contractions she asked if I wanted her to reach in and break the bulging bag of amniotic fluid. With my permission, she proceeded. Immediately I was on my hands and knees for my next 2 contractions as I brought my baby earthside. As I delivered my baby, my midwife said, "Pull your baby through your legs, Momma!" As I pulled baby up to my chest, I looked and there HE was! It was a BOY! After 26 hours of unmedicated labor, at 12:04pm on April 16, 2021. My second son, Jasper William.

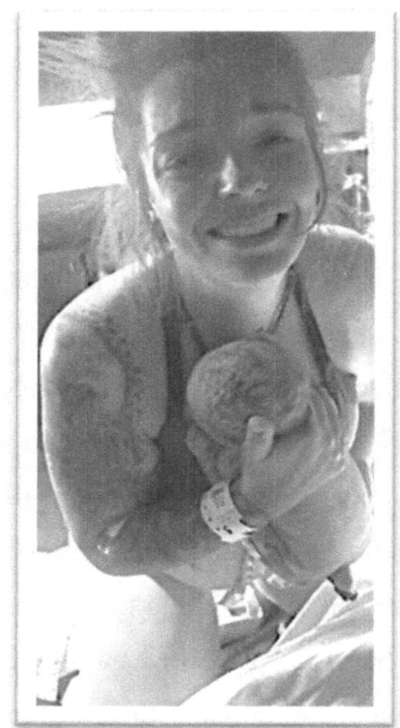

April 18, 2021

Mari, Ezra, and Ramona: A Twin Homebirth

My husband and I had two beautiful boys when we decided we wanted to try for one last baby. We found out we were pregnant and then that we were not expecting just one, but two babies. We had two previous home births and knew we wanted to try and have our twins at home, too. We found a doctor (which is required by law here) who would support our decision to birth at home. By 36 weeks I was ready for the babies to arrive. Every day waiting for them began to take its toll physically and emotionally.

On the morning of April 18th, at 38 weeks, I woke up around 4:30am feeling wet, as if I had peed my pants a little. I wasn't having any noticeable contractions, so I decided to try and go back to bed. I didn't want to get too excited in case this was a false alarm. At around 5:30 I noticed that I was continuing to leak fluid and felt like I might be having contractions. I decided to wake my husband at that point. By 6:00 I was pretty certain that I was in labor, so we called my mom to come pick up the boys and then phoned our midwife who would call the rest of the team and let them know to head over. I told my midwife she didn't need to rush.

At 7:00am I wanted to get in the bath, so I went to give my boys a kiss before they headed off with my mom. My midwife and her team arrived right around this time. After I got into the bath I began to feel a lot more pressure. I was so focused on my breathing and just thinking about these two little people we were going to meet very soon. My contractions were never really painful. After about 30 minutes of being in the bath I began to feel an intense amount of pressure. My midwife asked if I wanted to get out of the bath and I decided that I did. I sat down on a birthing stool and felt like I needed to push. At

7:48 I pushed out our baby A in one or two pushes. I immediately brought him up to my chest and was overcome with joy. I lifted him up and was so happy to announce that we had another little boy.

A few minutes after our boy was born, I heard one of the midwives say there was blood. The mood changed in the room and everyone turned their focus to our remaining baby B. Baby B's heart was dropping slightly and our doctor felt it would be best to perform a breech extraction right away. We all agreed that it would be best to do that. I handed our baby boy to my husband and we went on with the extraction.

This was the hardest part of my birth. The procedure was very uncomfortable and all the while we were anxiously waiting to get this baby out. The doctor told the midwives to get oxygen ready for the baby and to be ready to resuscitate. It felt like hours waiting for our baby to be pulled out. Finally, at 8:12, the baby was out and placed directly on my chest. I held the baby close as the midwife gave breaths of oxygen. I knew this baby was going to be ok. After a few minutes I held up baby B and with tears announced that it was a girl!

April 24, 2021

Desiree and Lydia: A Birth in Arizona

I spent my pregnancy reading books, watching birth videos, and preparing for an unmedicated labor. With my first, after being scared into it, I was induced. I spent 6 hours on Pitocin without any pain only to get an epidural out of fear that it MIGHT hurt at some point. This time was different. I understood birth. I was confident. I was unafraid. I was excited and I was ready. On April 23rd at 40 weeks and 2 days pregnant, I woke up and for the first time felt that it was okay if baby didn't come today. I was at peace. Planning a homebirth meant all my energy recently had gone into maintaining a perfectly clean house because I was convinced I'd feel embarrassed if my perfectly put together birth team saw how out of control my house can get.

This day I decided to put it all off until tomorrow. I'd been having some pain in my hip all day but wrote it off as typical end of pregnancy discomfort. At 6:00pm I went to the bathroom and saw my mucus plug, streaked with blood. I knew this meant it could be now or days from now, but that didn't stop the excitement. My body was doing things! At 7:30pm I sat to play a game with my husband and mom. I noticed that the hip pain was now coming and going with some small contractions. There was still no pain, just a different intensity. I thought it was nothing, but timed some anyway. It was consistent. When the game finished, I went to kiss my 2-year-old goodnight one final time. I started sobbing. This was my "ah-ha" moment. This is when my heart knew I was in labor. I knew that when he woke up, he wouldn't be my only baby anymore. I loved on my first baby for a moment before heading for the shower around 9:30pm.

In the shower I had my first "real" contraction. It was like the cramp before the worst diarrhea of your life that makes you beg to make it stop. I was absolutely convinced that this was not real labor because I was able to speak through contractions. I thought because I wasn't feeling like I was dying in pain, it wasn't "real labor." I could still talk through it and move around, so I finished my shower and laid on my left side thinking this would fizzle out. At 10:30pm I was timing contractions lasting 50 seconds every 4-5 minutes. I called my doula and she listened to me have two contractions and told me she'd call my team for me and call me back. She called back at 11:32pm and I was in the middle of the most intense contraction yet, so my husband answered. As I was groaning through the pressure, I heard her say,

"You need to get that tub set up now. We will all be there in 25 minutes."

In between contractions I helped set up my birthing space. I stopped often to breathe through the waves. My team arrived at 12:15am. My two midwives and my doula walked into my home and I felt an intense wave of emotions rush over me, somewhere between peace and panic. At this point I told my mom to contact my photographer (who lived 2 hours away) while we filled up the tub. My doula sensed my emotions and hugged me deeply. My midwife offered to check me. Wanting the reassurance that this was real and wasn't going to stop, I agreed. I was already 8 centimeters! I was seeking reassurance and I got it. It had been 3 hours since my first "real" contraction and I was already at an 8! I was doing it! This wasn't so bad! This was not the pain they warn you about! This was easy!

Before getting in the tub, my doula stood behind me and did belly lifts. I could feel my baby moving down into my pelvis with each contraction. It felt intense - emotionally and physically. I got in the tub and just sat, allowing the water to offer relief. I chatted with my midwives and held my husband's hand through the waves. This is when the night gets blurry. This is when it went from easy to hard work.

My contractions ramped up fast and I found myself struggling to find the low moans I was searching for. I was holding my breath and getting a bit panicky. This is when I completely lost my bearings. I knew in my heart I was in transition, but I couldn't formulate the thought or tell anyone what I needed. I was struggling. My midwife came over and very sternly told me I was breathing for my baby too, and I needed to focus on that. I tried. I found myself fighting against my contractions. I could not find my footing. I continued fighting my contractions by pulling away from the pain and pressure.

My doula asked me if I would feel steadier outside of the tub. At this point I would have agreed to anything. I was needing guidance and I trusted my team. The water was definitely too hot for me and I just couldn't find the stability I was searching for. I said yes, and she and my husband got me out of the tub. As she dried me off, she whispered, "It won't get any worse than this, baby. This is as bad as it gets." I didn't believe her. In hindsight, she was right.

As I crawled into my bed I glanced at my midwife's tablet and it said 1:07am. I remember being impressed with how quickly this was moving. I instinctively crawled onto my back - the last position I thought I'd want to be in, but the only place I felt stable. My midwives and doula recognized that I was not in tune with my body or my emotions so they guided me in pushing. I screamed. I wasn't the quiet woman pushing her baby out peacefully in the tub. I was roaring, I was high pitched, I was grunting. I was telling them I couldn't do it. I was struggling to not pull away from the pain, and repeatedly apologizing to no one in particular about all of it. Absolutely overwhelmed by the intensity of labor and pushing I told my husband, "I can't do this." He whispered in my ear, "You already are." Which is exactly what I needed to snap me back into my body.

I asked, "Am I sucking her back in?" My midwives giggled and said no, I was doing great. They assured me that they could see her bag of water and her dark hair floating inside. With each contraction I screamed and I pushed and I watched my midwife handing off little bits of toilet paper to be flushed. My waters broke as my daughter's head emerged. While there, she started to cry. That was it, that was the motivation I needed. I pushed once, her shoulders came out, pushed again and got to her belly. One final push and she was passed between my legs and onto my chest.

At 1:23am on April 24, 2021, Lydia Ray was born. My sweet rainbow. After just 4 hours. Four hours. My photographer arrived minutes after Lydia made her entrance. We waited calmly and patiently for my placenta. There was no rush. Forty-two minutes later I pushed my placenta out and started to bleed a bit more than the midwives liked. They gave me a tincture under my tongue to help regulate the bleeding. That seemed to do the trick. The magic of midwifery. While my husband and I loved on our newest member, my birth team cleaned up the "evidence," got me a snack, and helped me to the bathroom. After our skin to skin, the newborn exam was done at the foot of the bed. She weighed 8 pounds 10 ounces. After we were tucked into our fresh sheets, our team packed up and headed home. Our 2-year-old woke up to the sweet surprise of his baby sister being home. And I was in heaven. I had a homebirth! I had done something I thought was crazy three years prior during my first pregnancy. Was it the quiet, calm, completely in-tune with my body, incredible birth I thought it would be?

No.

It was the loud, raw, overwhelmingly intense, absolutely incredible birth, in a messy home with undone dinner dishes, that I needed it to be. Birth is magic.

April 25, 2021

Emily and Alora: A Birth in Texas

On Saturday, April 24th, I started having consistent contractions. They lasted most of the day but didn't gain intensity. We went to sleep and I woke up in the middle of the night to more contractions. They were more intense than the day before, so I figured this was probably labor. I slept in between contractions until I couldn't lay down anymore. Around 5:00am I got into the shower and woke up my husband. I texted my midwife to inform her that labor had started. After using the bathroom, I noticed my mucus plug and was kind of thrown off.

This labor was drastically different from my last two. I don't know if it felt slower because of me being more in tune with my body, or if it was because this labor was just slower. I texted my mom to come over - it was baby time! Just as she got here my labor started to intensify. I was kneeling and breathing through contractions and told my husband to fill up the tub. We had not practiced connecting the hose to the shower, so he and my mom tried to figure it out while I commanded them to hurry up. Finally, they figured it out and I hopped in the pool as it was being filled up. Just like during my last labor, the water was soothing and relieved the intensity of contractions.

Our older kiddos were awake at this point and pretty much stayed in the back of the house with my mom and sister. My midwife and her assistant arrived. As my baby was descending, I started to get tired. For a moment I could feel my confidence dwindling. I repeated affirmations to myself quietly. My husband put on music and lit an incense. This was my initiation, I needed to surrender. As I relinquished control, I could feel my baby crowning. As she was peacefully born into the water, my midwife guided her to my hands. Emotions overcame me as I placed our baby on my chest. She was covered in vernix.

We had decided to wait until birth to find out if baby was a boy or girl. My mom, sister, and kids came into the living room to meet their new sibling. I peeked to see if baby number four was a boy or girl. "GIRL!" I exclaimed. We allowed Alora to stay connected to the placenta for some time. After the birth of the placenta - we clamped, cut the cord, and passed her to daddy for skin to skin. My midwife helped me out of the tub and into the shower.

As I was showering, my midwife checked for tearing. No tearing! I passed several clots, thankfully in the normal size range. While I showered, my midwife and her assistant changed the sheets, emptied the birth pool, and started a load of laundry.

After showering they helped me into bed and my husband handed Alora back to try and breastfeed. The kids took turns holding their new baby sister. It was important for me to have them at the birth so they could witness a natural life event. We chatted about the series of events and all of the newborn procedures took place at the bottom of the bed. It was so nice knowing we were in the comfort of our home and didn't have to go anywhere. Alora's birth was about 7 hours. It was serene and magical. Home birth was everything I desired and more!

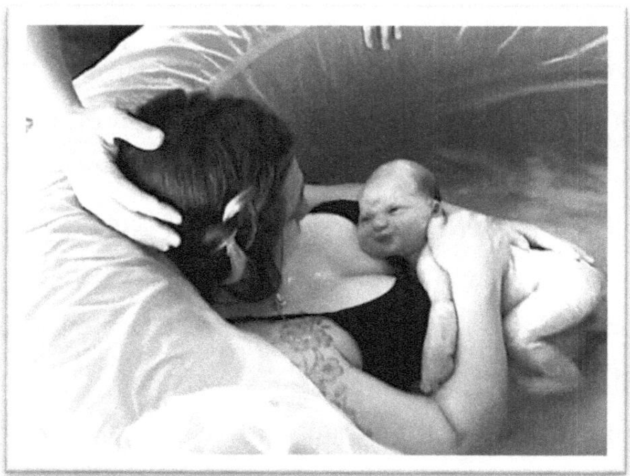

Adriana and Shea Violet

It was Sunday, April 25th, when I finally went into labor. I woke up that morning disappointed again because I hadn't gone into labor overnight. I know that staying relaxed and calm is supposed to help, but when you're 5 days past your due date, with a 19-month-old and still going to work, it's hard. I had been doing everything to get things moving, so when my husband wiggled his eyebrows at me when it was naptime for the toddler, I thought "Why not?" I had laid there for a while when I felt the first contraction. I figured it was only because we had just had sex and that they would taper off, but I was wrong. About an hour later I mentioned to my husband that I thought we were going to have a baby that day. I was breathing through the contractions easily at this point, ready to finally give birth.

It was now about 5:00pm and I had been laboring since 12:30. I decided to call the doctor to let them know I was in labor and ask if I should come to the hospital yet. I had been tracking my contractions and they were about a minute long and 5 minutes apart but had only been that way for 25 minutes or so. I live about 35 minutes from the hospital. The doctor said I could come in, so we started packing up the car to get ready to leave. The car ride was bumpy and uncomfortable. I was still breathing through the contractions, but they were becoming more and more intense and I didn't like not being able to move around and shift positions.

We finally got to the hospital around 6:00 and were taken upstairs pretty quickly to triage, where I had my cervix checked. I was so discouraged hearing that I was only 4 centimeters dilated. I had been walking around at 3 centimeters and 75% effaced for two weeks prior, so I thought that I would at least be 5 or 6 centimeters by the time I was in active labor. I also got the dreaded COVID swab, and was so thankful that it came back negative and I could labor without my mask on.

I met my nurse and student nurse (who was previously a doula- I was very excited about this) and quickly went over with them what I wanted for my birth. I immediately said no more students, no epidural, low intervention, intermittent monitoring, use of the shower, and possibly nitrous if I felt like I needed it. The student nurse showed my husband how to do counter pressure, and then they left.

After everyone was out of the room, I immediately got into the shower. I was having pretty bad back labor, so my husband used the handheld showerhead and kept the warm water flowing over my lower back. I remember swaying and moaning with each contraction. I tried to remember to keep my body and face relaxed and used the water to keep me distracted. I had been in the shower for a while when I told my husband I felt like I needed to lay down to relax and try the nitrous. My RN got everything set up and the doctor came in to tell me how to use it. I breathed through a couple contractions using it and it made me feel a little loopy, but it didn't take much of the pain away - and it made me nauseous. While I was laying down my midwife decided to check my cervix. Now I was 7 centimeters and into transition. She asked if she could break my water and I declined.

After the cervical check I got back into the shower for a while. Then I got up on the hospital bed on my hands and knees. I'm not sure how much time went by, transition is like an out of body experience. My midwife wanted another cervical check and I was 9 centimeters. When the midwife asked again to break my water, this time I agreed, knowing that pushing was only a few minutes away anyway.

After my water was broken the contractions were extremely intense and I immediately wanted to get up to help ease the pain. I was kneeling on top of the bed using the squat bar with one leg up and one kneeling, kind of like a "proposing" position. I was rocking and swaying when my midwife and OB wanted to see if I was complete and ready to start pushing. They did request that I lay on my back because my baby was estimated to be on the larger side, which I think in hindsight wasn't the best decision for me, but when you're about to push out a baby you don't really have it in you to argue.

I got in position and started to push. And that's when her heart rate began to drop. I gave a few more pushes and then things started to get a little frantic. My OB told me, "We have to get her out NOW," and told me to push as hard as I could. In between contractions, I could feel their hands inside me. It hurt so bad to have their hands in there. When I got to the next contraction, I gave another good push. Then my OB said, "Ok I think we have to cut you to get her out." I knew that I didn't want that, but I would do anything to make sure my baby got here safely. Another contraction started and I pushed harder than I ever have and she came out in that one push.

Immediately she was placed on my chest, but it only felt like it was for a moment while they cut the cord and then whisked her off to the warmer. She was purple when she came out but she pinked up and gave a good cry when they began to rub her with the blankets. Once they deemed her healthy, they brought her back to me to do skin to skin. She latched almost immediately and it was one of the best feelings in the entire world. She was perfect. I felt so triumphant with her birth, even though not everything went exactly as planned.

Abby and Penelope: A Birth in New Hampshire

On April 29th, at 3:35pm, I had my second daughter in my arms. That morning, at almost 42 weeks pregnant, I woke up feeling like it was going to be the day. The day before I had a lot of overwhelming emotions during a visit with my dear friend and doula, Tia. I swore I couldn't keep going on being pregnant. I was actually letting myself go to a place where I contemplated getting induced if she didn't come by the end of the weekend. I was just so done with being pregnant. I was contracting daily but it would always fizzle out. Mike kept missing out on work. I was slipping into a state of depression and anxiety. Not to mention, constantly finding childcare for Lyla, so I could get into my wild brain for labor to progress. I was at my breaking point - or so I thought.

Later that night I was able to reach a state of peace. I no longer felt I was done, and I didn't feel the need to rush this little girl of mine. I felt she would come when she was ready and that this was her first lesson for me. I went to bed at peace and happy knowing I trusted my body and I trusted my baby to choose the perfect time to be born. There was a plan in place and it wasn't my plan to make.

The next morning, I woke up around 7:30 and got up to use the bathroom. Something felt different. It felt just how it did the morning I went into labor with my older daughter, Lyla. I just knew it was the day. I looked at Mike and he knew it too. Of course, we had trees being taken down in our yard with an entire tree crew outside. That is just how life works, right?

Around 8:00am my contractions started rolling in. I let them roll in and phase out. I surrendered to what was happening and released all control and trust over to my body and my baby. After about an hour of contractions, I told Mike to make the necessary phone calls. While Mike got ahold of my mom, Tia and got Lyla to the neighbor's house, I labored in the bath tub upstairs. I was able to be in my own space and let my body do what it was made to do. When my mom arrived and Lyla was all set next door playing with the kids and having a great time, I was able to fully let go. My mom suggested a walk to keep things moving.

I felt it was a good time to reach out to our midwife and let her know I was having contractions for the last two hours at 7 minutes apart. I noticed I had a voice mail from her, so I listened to it first. She was telling me that because I was nearly 42 weeks, if my baby didn't come before the end of the weekend we needed to come up with a new plan and consider induction. I called her back immediately and told her I was in labor. She asked me if I wanted to have some castor oil to pick things up. I quickly refused and told her I would prefer to let me body do this on its own. She told me to contact her if things picked up.

We set out to walk around the neighborhood. I couldn't walk more than a couple feet without having a contraction, but at this point I was still laughing and joking between them. The normally fifteen-minute walk took us an hour to complete, and Tia arrived right as we got back home. We all went back into the house and Tia suggested I try and eat something while I could. I was able to get down a peanut butter sandwich and then decided I should rest. I wanted to gather all my strength for what was to come.

I laid up in my bed, which was one of the best parts about planning a home birth. I had my mom come up with me while Mike started filling the birth pool. Then they switched and Mike rubbed my back while I let the contractions come and go in the comfort of my bedroom. Then something didn't feel right. I was told by Tia during my whole pregnancy that I would know before anyone if something wasn't right during the birth. She was right. Mike and I headed down stairs to where her and my mom were. The contractions kept coming, and at this point they were all in my back. With each wave came a swift kick into my tailbone that made me feel like I was being sucker punched from the inside and paralyzed. It was excruciating. I remember saying to Tia, "Something isn't right. I never felt this with Lyla. We need to change her position." Tia agreed and had me get down on all fours and do some stretches to help reposition Penelope. We also did some work with the rebozo.

Luckily this helped. After riding out a few contractions while holding these positions, the back labor stopped. Now that we got her into a better position, contractions were coming faster and more frequent. Up until this point my contractions had been consistently 5-7 minutes apart and they changed to 2-3 minutes apart. They continued like that for another hour and then they slowed down and I rested.

I let my body surrender to this next stage of labor. I was in a blissful state where no one could reach me. Tia tried to get my attention and suggested I try moving my body to help things progress as they all thought things were slowing down. When I gently whispered, "No, I need to rest." Tia jumped into action and quickly remembered this from Lyla's birth with me. That's when she knew. She told Mike to call the midwife again and to finish filling up the birth pool. As soon as Mike got back, Tia suggested we make our way downstairs into the basement where the birth pool and space was set up. I suggested I use the bathroom first.

I moved to the bathroom and had four major contractions. The way they felt, the way I sounded, it was all so different than what was happening before. Tia reassured us that by now it was 3:00pm and the midwife should arrive soon. She made sure I was reminded that this was all normal and my body and my baby were working together and I was fully capable of this hard work.

As we made our way down the stairs, which took about 20 minutes, I had three more huge contractions. I made my way over to the birth pool and was helped while I got in. To my surprise, almost immediately as my pelvis touched the water, I realized that whole time I had been in transition. I had now entered the fetal ejection reflex stage of labor. There was no more control over my body, my breath, or my contractions. My body took over completely and my baby was ready to enter the world. At this point, the midwife was not at the house and it was still just the 4, soon to be 5 of us. I didn't have time to think or even notice. Within minutes my contractions were pushes and it was so instinctual.

My contractions were lasting much longer and were so much more intense. My second contraction in the birth pool and I couldn't believe it, Penelope's head was crowning. No one could believe it. None of us thought I was THIS close. I screamed "Her head, her head!" They didn't believe me until Tia looked and reassured me, I was safe and so was my baby. Her head was emerging. Then the third contraction came and I roared like a wild animal, but she was regressing back in. That is when I knew something was holding her back.

I was scared, but I didn't have time to be scared. I just yelled, "She's stuck, she's stuck, she's not coming!"

Tia reassured me I knew what to do and to calm my body and my breath. To just breathe. I took deep breathes as I held my baby's head. I didn't know what to do. How could I? This is what I had hired a midwife for. Then my instinct kicked in and I reached in and felt the cord wrapped around her shoulder which was keeping her from progressing. I felt the next contraction building and when it hit, I moved the cord out of the way and screamed. I used every strength within me and pushed my baby out. She came flying out once her cord was moved out of her way. As soon as she was out, I unraveled the cord from her shoulder and I placed her on my chest. I felt the immediate relief and state of euphoric bliss I longed for. I did it. She was out. She was alive, I was alive, and we were both safe.

As I was sitting in the birth pool with my newly born daughter on my chest and my placenta still not birthed, I realized my midwife was still not there. My first words to everyone were, "Where the F is the midwife?"

Did that really just happen? That really just happened. We waited for what felt like an eternity, but was actually about twenty minutes, before the midwife's assistant showed up. She got me and Penelope out of the pool and on the couch where she assisted me in birthing the placenta. It was such a relief to have it out. I felt like I could completely breathe now.

At 4:15pm, the midwife had finally arrived and checked us both out to make sure our vitals were good. She then told me I would need stitches and I asked if they were necessary. She assured me they were. As she gave me a lidocaine injection and had her assistant start suturing, I told them that the injection didn't numb me, I could feel it. This was not the first time I had stitches after birth and I knew it wasn't supposed to feel this way. She gave me another injection which burned and I was sobbing at this point. I just wanted to enjoy my baby. I didn't want to go through anything else. Again, I could feel it all. She proceeded to give me a third injection as I was still sobbing and begging her to just stop and not do any more. She told me she had to, which is not true. I let her, I cried the whole time and gripped my mother's hands so hard while I watched my husband squirm while watching and holding our newly born daughter. After the stitches were done, I wanted nothing to do with the midwife. I was so disgusted by the care I received from her. Her not showing up at my birth and then to treat me that way post-birth. I just wanted to be in my bed with my baby.

My mom and Tia got me up and the nurse who came checked me out again and helped me get dressed. I came upstairs to the couch and was handed my baby - she was finally back in my arms. Once I had my second baby in my arms, I instantly needed my first. I begged my father who had arrived moments before, to go grab her from the neighbor's so we could have her meet her new baby sister. This moment was one of the best moments of my life. The way her eyes lit up when she saw her sister for the first time was the best thing I've ever seen. She smiled so big and said, "My baby!" She instantly came over and hugged and kissed her and climbed up on my lap and I had both of my babies with me.

My story doesn't end here. I may have had a birth for the books, but I ended up suffering majorly with PPD, I had birth trauma I had to work through, a shocked nervous system that needed repairing and I needed a lot more help with two under two than I anticipated. The postpartum period is part of it. A home birth was such an incredible experience, one I wouldn't trade for anything. What a unique story Penelope will have and what a remarkable story I get to tell and to hold on to on my hardest days. I did that. I birthed my baby. I birthed her based on instinct and the support of my closest support, the support that carried me through Lyla's birth as well. My team. The people in my life I consider my best friends. I did that.

May

May 2, 2021

Summer and River: A Birth in California

To River Phoenix,

Here is your birth story for you to have and share...

Let's start with the couple of days before I had you. Your dad was on a brush fire up in Castaic, California, which is about 2 hours away from where we live in Murrieta. I was worried I would go into labor and he wouldn't make it home in time. Fortunately, Daddy's captain was able to get him off the fire and he came home on April 30th. As soon as your dad came home, we went to go get an acupressure massage. I told them that you were overdue and I wanted to go into labor. We were getting so anxious to meet you. After that we had our final lunch as a family of two. I kept talking about the midwives' brew and how other people have taken it to help get them in labor, but I was nervous about drinking castor oil. I texted my Aunt Deb (a midwife) and she said it was fine.

At 5:30pm on April 30th, I drank 2 tablespoons of castor oil mixed in with a protein shake. It was actually delicious. Thirty minutes after that I started to feel small contractions and some cramping. Your dad and I sat on the couch and watched Netflix until I was ready to go to bed. As I was watching Netflix, I started crying at the thought of going into labor and meeting you. Right before bed, your dad asked me when my water would break or when that usually happens. I laughed at him and told him that only really happens in the movies and it probably wouldn't break until after I got to the hospital. When I went to bed, my contractions and the cramping didn't allow me to sleep. I kept tossing and turning and getting up to go to pee. At 3:00am I got up to go pee again and as I was walking to the bathroom, I felt a slow trickle down my leg that didn't stop. MY WATER BROKE! I woke your dad up and started crying. You were officially on your way. I called my midwife who was on call at the time and she said I had to be at the hospital in 12 hours. I asked your dad if we could just get a hotel so that I could labor there until I was ready to get to the hospital. As we left the house, the contractions started getting stronger and more uncomfortable. We left to head to Irvine, California.

We checked into our hotel and the contractions kept building. I was unable to lay in bed during them anymore. I called my doula, Kristen, and let her know it was getting close and she should probably come. She arrived around 8:45am and I decided I really needed to try and get some rest. I laid down in the bed and fell asleep and unfortunately the contractions had stopped. After a short nap, we began walking laps around the hotel and going up and down the stairs to hopefully jump start labor. By 1:00pm I needed to get to the hospital to make sure that you were still doing okay - my water had been broken for almost 10 hours now. When I called the midwife on call, she said the hospital was really full and there wasn't a midwife birthing suite open and to call back in an hour. When I called back, she said to come around 2:30pm and that she would find a room for me. Your dad and Kristen helped me do some curb walking to burn time and hopefully start labor again, but it didn't help.

We got to the hospital and checked into triage. The midwife, Jessica, told me that I could try pumping to get labor started again. While I was in triage, I pumped over 10 milliliters of colostrum. I was beyond excited that I was starting to make milk for you! Sure enough, the contractions started shortly after that but kept stopping as soon as I stopped pumping. She told us to go out to the meditation garden and try doing some squats and lunges to start labor. Your dad had me working out outside. The one thing that seemed to help the most was high knees. After thirty minutes of working out, the nurse came and got me and took me back to have Jessica check my progress. I was 90% effaced and 2-3 centimeters dilated. She was able to strip my membranes. We were then taken back to our midwife suite. These suites were made for women who want to have a natural, physiological birth. It literally looked like I was walking into a 5-star hotel. There was a huge queen size bed, a rocking chair, a rainfall shower to labor in, and a blow-up bath tub. Labor wasn't progressing so I tried pumping some more. I was getting really discouraged that my labor wasn't ever going to start and that I would need Pitocin, but Jessica reassured me that I wasn't going to get anything I didn't want.

After a few hours of trying to get labor going via pumping and going back and forth between our hospital room and the meditation garden, Jessica sat me down and asked me what I wanted to do. I told her I was really tired because I didn't' sleep the night before. She told me that I should probably rest and that maybe my labor would start. Your dad and I got into bed around 10:00 and were snuggling when the contractions started at 11:00. I was never able to fall asleep. Jessica then began to fill the tub up with warm water for me to labor in since they were getting really uncomfortable. I sat in that tub for hours and every contraction, your dad coached me through my breathing. I was getting exhausted and began to fall asleep in between each contraction. I actually fell asleep and my head dunked under the water. I scared everyone for a second.

Every contraction required me to get on my hands and knees to handle the discomfort, I was getting tired of holding myself up in the water and your poor dads back probably felt like it was going to break because he was supporting my weight during the contractions. Your dad is the most patient and kind person. The pain became so unbearable that I threw up and requested to get out of the water and into bed and try some nitrous oxide to relieve the pain. They set up the machine for me which required me to put this mask on my face and breath through it when a contraction was starting. Your dad kept trying to get me to take one regular breath and one then one nitrous oxide breath. He was worried I was going to get too much of it or hyperventilate. I literally told him, "I am going to fuck you up," when he tried to take it away. (The staff all laughed at this later). At this point the contractions were right on top of each other and I was beginning to question my strength and ability to have a natural birth.

I asked your dad about getting a shot of Stadol to help with the pain. He told me that I was too strong and that I would be disappointed in myself if I took it. I begged him for it. The midwife came in to check on me, after stepping out only for a short period of time, and I asked her about a pain shot. She said that would require me to get on the monitors (which I hadn't had to do this entire time). I told her never mind because I didn't want to be connected to anything. She reminded me of how strong I was and that I could do this. She sat behind me and began rubbing my back and giving me a massage to help me with the pain. The midwives were literally incredible. They were so patient and kind. They were in the room for hours with me just sitting there helping in any way I needed.

After a while of laboring in bed, she checked me and said I had a lip on my cervix that the baby was stuck on and then told me I should probably go and get onto the toilet and labor there for a bit. I was resistant to leaving my nitrous oxide, but it didn't seem to be helping. I went to the bathroom and switched off between the shower and sitting on the toilet. Don't resist the toilet - it surprisingly seemed to really help me. When I was in the shower your dad took the shower head and sprayed me and coached me through every contraction.

After pushing on the toilet for a bit, the midwives moved me to a squatting chair where your dad sat behind me and held me through every contraction. I reached down and could feel your head. This gave me so much motivation to push harder. The burning became so unreal I started crying, "Ring of fire!" Your dad had no clue what that meant. Your head was almost out and one midwife coached me to slow down and let your head turn so that you could come out. After a few pushes they told me to reach down and grab you. Your dad supported my full body weight, I pushed as hard as I could and then reached down and grabbed you. You were turned around so all your dad and I could see was your back. I flipped you over and said, "It's a boy!" Your dad and I began crying!

The feeling was unreal. Fifteen hours of excruciating pain was over. You made me a mama at 7:45am on May 2, 2021. You weighed 7 pounds, 11 ounces and were 19 inches long. The midwives and your dad helped get me back to bed and you laid on my chest while they helped deliver my placenta. They also sewed up my labial tear. Funny little story, the suturing was painful, and I wasn't paying attention, but I needed to grab on to someone's hand to squeeze. Well, it turns out I was squeezing your hand for comfort and your dad said, "Babe that's his little hand." You didn't complain at all. After my delivery team left the room, your dad and I laid in bed with you and snuggled. You fell asleep on your dad's chest while I closed my eyes. We were so exhausted from being up for over thirty hours.

And that is the story of how you were born. You'll never know how much I love you for making me a mom. You're absolutely perfect.

May 4, 2021

Krystal and Elias

On May 4th, we welcomed our son earthside. My water broke at 3:35am and I started getting contractions about an hour after. I labored at home until about 1:30pm and labored in the car for an hour on the way to the birth center. We arrived at the birth center at 2:30 in the afternoon. I consented to a cervical check and was 7 centimeters dilated. Within thirty minutes (I think), I immediately felt the overwhelming urge to push. The midwives and my doula encouraged me to listen to my body the entire time. I pushed for almost 5 hours! I labored and pushed in the tub, on the toilet, on my hands and knees, and in a side lying position. I had an anterior cervical lip that my midwife tried to push out of the way after going into the reset position for a while, but it got swollen. I eventually pushed past it. He was in the right occiput posterior position (sunny side up) for most of my labor, and he was having a difficult time descending.

At 8:00pm, my midwife came up with two plans. Plan A was to try and squat him out (which I hadn't really been doing). Then if that didn't work, Plan B was to transfer to a hospital to get an epidural so that I could get some rest. I literally could not stop pushing! After I heard Plan B, I knew I had to get him out ASAP! I pushed in a squat and then we saw his head! I pushed for another twenty minutes, and he was here! My husband caught him and immediately placed him in my arms.

May 15, 2021

Monica and Ocean

I started having light contractions at 3:00am on Saturday morning. I had not slept yet so I tried to go to sleep quickly since I knew I would soon need as much energy as I could get. I napped for three hours before waking up to a contraction. It wasn't painful at all but was too hard to sleep through, so I got up. I made my celery juice and protein smoothie bowl and texted my doula. I didn't want my midwife or doula to be here longer than they needed to, so I spent the entire day logging my contractions on my Ovia app, waiting for them to be 5-1-1 (Five minutes apart, one minute long, and continuing for one hour.) This is when I'd call my doula. I would call my midwife when the contractions got to a pattern of 4-1-1.

At 7:00pm my husband told me to call my doula, Lexi. I told him I was supposed to call when my contractions were 5 minutes apart for an hour and I wasn't there yet. He still made me call, but since he was in another room, I told her that I felt fine and I was just calling because he wanted me to. I even ended the call saying, "Take your time!" My midwife called me soon after for an update and after I told her I felt everything in my back, she told me to do the Miles Circuit. I googled it and was trying to figure it out while at the same time my contractions got more intense and closer together.

My doula arrived at 8:00, right as I realized my contractions were only two minutes apart. I remember I kept saying, "I just want to go to the bathroom." Lexi informed me that I would feel this need the entire time, so I gave up on that and told her that the midwife wanted me to do the Miles Circuit. She had me lay in one of the positions for three contractions while Jon finished filling the birthing pool. My water still hadn't broken and I was worried that I would miss that if I was in the water, but at this point the pain in my back was so intense. I got in the water as soon as we finished the exercise. Almost immediately my body took over. I didn't push, but my body did. Just like hiccups, I couldn't control it. During these "hiccups" I felt like my back was going to break. Lexi kept rubbing my lower back and it felt so good and reassuring to have her there. On my third "hiccup" I felt his head pass through and heard, "Her water just broke!"

Lexi and Jon saw the head. Jon hopped in the pool immediately, not even having enough time to take off his shirt. My doula had my midwife on the speaker phone, and she kept saying to push with my next contraction. I couldn't figure out how to push since my body did it for me before. I tried to breathe my baby down like I learned about in hypnobirthing classes and then let out a large groan. On my next contraction, at 8:56pm, the rest of Ocean Kingston came out into Jon's arms while "Here Comes the Sun" by the Beatles played in the background. My midwife arrived shortly after to assist in the birth of the placenta. She was so helpful after birth. I am so incredibly grateful to my birth team for allowing me to have my perfect birth.

When I found out I was pregnant, I educated myself with books, statistics, classes, and documentaries on birth. Many people have called me "brave" for having a home birth. I am not brave. I just knew all of my options and chose what was best for me and my baby.

May 18, 2021

Christina and Eleanor: A Birth in Illinois

I'd been struggling with preterm labor issues for weeks. Twice I had spent the night at the hospital, getting medication to help stop contractions and to monitor me and my daughter. The first time was at 28 weeks and the second time was at 33 weeks and 5 days. I remember that so specifically because had it been 2 days later and I was 34 weeks, the doctor would have just let me have her. I also had the worst back pain I'd ever experienced in the weeks leading up to giving birth. Everyone told me that it was back labor, but I didn't completely believe that.

On May 18th, I went to my doctor for my weekly checkup and was told that I was dilated to 4 centimeters and was very thin. He said that it wouldn't be long at all before I had her, and he had me schedule an ultrasound appointment for the next day. At this point I was 35 weeks and limping from the pain in my back. The wonderful feeling of pregnancy was gone and I was ready to be done.

My husband and I left the doctor's office at 3:00pm and went to lay in our bed for a bit. Around 5:00 I woke up free of pain - I truly felt the best I'd felt in over a month! We went to the store to get some random odds and ends when I very suddenly felt intense cramps. I went to the bathroom hoping that was the issue, but they just kept getting worse and worse. We left the store and by the time we got home the contractions, which I still thought were just cramps, had turned into one long, continuous pain.

I walked, squatted, and crawled at home until nearly 8:00pm. Finally, my husband made the call that we should go to the hospital. It was definitely the right call. We got there just after 9:00pm and my water had been leaking all day without me noticing. I was 9 centimeters dilated and I went straight into the delivery room. I had to wait for the doctor to get there. He walked in and, according to my husband, my daughter arrived less than 10 minutes later. A beautiful, 5 pounds 9 ounces, 18.5 inch little girl with a head full of hair was born.

May 20, 2021

Maria and Wesley

My first contractions started on May 18th around 11:30pm. I'd had Braxton hicks often, but these were VERY different. So I texted my doula and we synced on an app so she could see me time my contractions through a live stream. She suggested I take a warm bath/shower because my contractions weren't very consistent. This continued through the entire night, resulting in me getting maybe 2 hours of sleep total in between the contractions. She helped me get an appointment with a chiropractor for the following day. By this point my contractions were still all over the place. I had a tilted pelvis and my pubic bone was not aligned so the baby wasn't engaging well. The chiropractor fixed me up. I then headed down the road to my midwife's office for a quick check in. She said I was almost 5 centimeters dilated. I went home and things started to pick up.

I took another hot bath and tried to rest with no luck. My doula headed over to help me work through my contractions. They were getting stronger, but were not consistent. I continued to try sleeping and sitting on my yoga ball. Around midnight, I got into a hot bath again and managed to doze off. My contractions really picked up and were back-to-back like waves. I got out of the tub and headed to my living room, feeling the urge to push. We had the birth pool set up but no hot water because I had used it all by filling the bathtub. My mom went to try filling it with water from her side of the house. We called her back telling her it was too late and it was time.

My midwife was still on her way and I had no choice but to go with the flow. My doula, who also happens to be a midwife apprentice, got into baby catching mode just in case. My midwife got there soon after and I leaned back on my couch to rest. They checked me and noticed my baby was definitely ready to be born. I dozed in and out of sleep in between contractions for a while. I was in transition, and I felt so sleepy and exhausted, like I couldn't even move.

Suddenly, I was hit with the strongest contractions. My birth team suggested that Noel pull one end of a rebozo and we do a tug-of-war technique. I scrounged up the last burst of energy I had. I went into a deep squat and screamed and groaned. All I felt was a huge gush and a release of pressure. One of the midwives was splashed with the amniotic fluid when my water broke. Then I felt the dreaded "ring of fire." I let out one more roar and my baby's head was out. My mom was cheering me on saying, "I see his face, keep going!" My husband and everyone cheered me on to keep pushing. I went into another squat and let my entire weight go on the rebozo. My poor husband held my entire weight on the other end, resulting in him popping three ribs out of place.

As soon as I squatted, I got back onto the edge of my couch. One of the midwife apprentices was massaging the top of my belly to help the baby out and I remember saying, "Wait. Give me a minute." As soon as she let go, baby Wesley Noel flew out without a single push! Luckily, my midwife was right there and caught him. I instantly reached out to hold him. My three older children came in to meet their brother and we've all been in love with him ever since. It was such a magical moment.

May 26, 2021

Zoha and Nusaybah

I had a traumatic birth with my first kiddo in 2018. After an epidural, stalled labor, and two hours of pushing, I was taken for a cesarean. My hemoglobin dropped from 14 to 4 and because my baby was already in the birth canal they had to push him back up and ripped my cervix in the process. I was in the hospital for a week after birth. This experience made me "high risk" for future pregnancies.

I started trying to have my second child but struggled with infertility while searching for a doctor. I eventually found one I liked who helped me get pregnant. First I reached out to midwives because I was so traumatized from the hospital birth, but they said I was too high risk for them to take me into their care. I finally found a doctor who I liked. She was cooperative and she listened to me. I also made sure to hire a doula this time. We had some issues that required regular monitoring towards the end of pregnancy and I was told the baby had a growth restriction so they wanted to induce me.

I got my praying hands out because I wanted a natural birth without medicine. I believe the epidural played a role in my previous c-section. I prayed that if induction was best for me and my baby, that's what would happen, and if not to make something better happen. I went into labor 24 hours before I was supposed to be induced. I went to the hospital when my contractions were 2 minutes apart. My labor stalled at the hospital a bit because I was stressed. Being back in the same environment as my first birth trauma was difficult. My doula suggested getting some medicine that would help me nap for an hour since I hadn't slept well all week.

We got a nap in and around 1:00pm active labor began. I thought I might not make it without pain medicine, but at 2:45 the nurse and doctor said that my water bag was out of my cervix and if they broke it, I could start pushing. I was on my knees on the bed and was told I was pushing well but I was exhausted. She said if I flipped over, she could check the position of the baby and see how to help. With the help of a vacuum, two pushes later my baby girl was born. She did skin to skin with me until I was sewn up. She was around 5 pounds and had some glucose and temperature issues, as well as some jaundice that she was hospitalized for.

My birth experience, even with baby girl's issues, was magical compared to the first. I could walk. I could pick my baby up. It was a healing experience for me.

May 28, 2021

Stefana

On May 28, 2021, at 5:30am, I woke up feeling some leaking. I went to the restroom and realized that I had lost my mucus plug and was leaking some fluid. I had been having irregular contractions for weeks, but this morning they were more frequent. I went about business as usual. I ate, drank some water, went for a walk, and showered. The contractions didn't go away. I definitely was in labor. My then 22-month-old son had no idea what was happening, which helped keep me distracted. We went for a long walk, and I would stop and get through each contraction. I heard that subsequent babies come faster, but my first was a very LONG labor - 54.5 hours. So I still didn't fully believe that this was really labor.

Around 1:00pm I ate some lunch and then very quickly got sick and threw it back up. The contractions were becoming stronger, and I was starting to not really want to talk very much. My husband thought it would be a good time to have the grandparents come and get my son and our dogs. I took what would be our last picture as a family of three with my baby boy, and off he went with grandma and papa. I was very emotional and knew he wouldn't be my baby anymore. How could I ever love another baby as much as I loved him?

I labored a bit longer and around 4:00pm my husband and I decided it was probably time to head to the hospital. I was still feeling a bit unsure of leaving and didn't realize how close together my contractions really were. I knew being at the hospital could slow my progress down and I wanted to get there just in time to push out our baby. We left and I felt contractions the whole ride to the hospital. When I got there, I couldn't even open my eyes. I could barely talk. I was holding one of my son's toy cars to remind me that I could get through the next contraction and soon I would be holding my baby.

I was taken up in a wheelchair and my husband checked us in. I labored in the waiting room for about an hour and a half before I was called in. I tried to peacefully get through each contraction. I made the mistake of giving up the wheelchair, and struggled to walk when I was called back. I could only get through a few steps before feeling the next contraction. The nurse just completely walked ahead of me, probably thinking I wasn't very far along. Then came all of the questions, the ones I was dreading because I knew that they would break my focus. But I got through them while my husband went and parked the car. I was in control of my labor, and I stayed relaxed through each contraction. I consented to a cervical check and to their surprise, I was 6 centimeters dilated. I remember looking at the clock and I was 6 centimeters at 6:00pm. Unfortunately, we checked in an hour before there was a shift change and we had new nurses within the right after we arrived.

124

The contractions were getting stronger. I felt a huge pop and my water had officially broken. Then the contractions got VERY strong. At this point I was asking for pain relief and my husband reminded me the epidural didn't work last time. I had asked him to help remind me of my birth goals during labor. He gently reminded me that I wanted to get our baby out without interventions. My OB asked if I was feeling "pushy" and I replied that I wasn't sure. My husband later told me that he knew I was ready. I went to the restroom and then went to lay down. Everyone had left the room except my husband. From the time that my OB asked me if I was feeling "pushy" to getting back in bed, it felt like only a minute. In that minute I went from being unsure if I was ready to push to, "OUR BABY IS COMING OUT RIGHT NOW!" I had this sudden urge to push.

My husband remained calm and was fully prepared to catch the baby if needed. I was yelling in pain as I felt him drop and start to crown. The nurses came rushing in and told me not to push yet, but I had no control over the pushing. My body was doing it for me. The pain seemed unbearable, but I had gotten this far and I knew he was close. My OB came in very calmly and ready to catch him. He came out so quickly, it felt like seconds. He was out in 2 pushes, but I didn't even "push," my body just did it. Then at 8:26pm I heard my beautiful 9 pound 15 ounce baby crying and he was placed on my chest. I immediately felt in complete shock of how quickly it seemed to happen and that I delivered unmedicated. I would do it all again in a heartbeat.

May 29, 2021

Kristen and Taylor

I was told my whole pregnancy that Taylor was measuring to be small - there was talk of moving our due date up and potentially having additional ultrasounds, but we opted to just wait and see. On May 29th, our estimated due date, I woke up at 4:30am because my water had broken! It was more of a steady trickle than a gush and continued throughout the day. I called the midwife, and she advised me to come in around 6:30 so they could check Taylor's vitals. All vitals looked good, and we made a plan to come back at 1:30pm to check again. We got breakfast and went home to watch Andy Griffith, walk around our neighborhood a few times, and do the Miles Circuit to see if contractions would pick up.

James went to get a haircut and put on a nice shirt and slacks. He wanted to make a good first impression when he met his daughter. The second vitals check was still good, but no contractions or active labor, so we planned to try a castor oil/almond butter/apricot juice cocktail if labor hadn't started by 4:30pm. We cuddled on the couch for a lot of the day, just relaxing and preparing. We took a long drive out in the country, looking at the scenery and watching the rain fall. By 6:30, I was having regular enough contractions to time them. After having them for an hour and them being strong enough that I was not able to talk or walk through them, James called the midwife. She suggested trying a warm bath. We tried and the contractions got stronger. It was time to go!

We arrived at the birth center around 8:30pm. At my first and only cervical check, I was dilated 7 centimeters. By the time I got into the pool, I felt like I was existing outside my own body. The contractions were so intense - and while my memory of this period is foggy, I know I bellowed and howled my way through them like a wild thing. I couldn't fight them, so I totally lost myself in the work my body was doing to bring my girl into the world.

When it was time for her to make her entrance, I was so drained. I told my mom and James, "I cannot do this." I felt my hands growing limp and weak and I couldn't keep my grip on the side of the pool to stay above the water. That's when James grabbed both of my hands and held them there. I remember him and my mom rubbing my back, giving me cold cloths, applying counter pressure to my hips, and telling me, "You can do this." But when I felt like I couldn't, they physically held me and kept me going.

Finally, I felt her coming and it was time to push. The first push delivered her head to her nose. The second push delivered her head. The third push brought her shoulders and body - the hard part was over, and she was in my arms. She gave one tiny little squeak of a cry before settling against me. She immediately knew to try to nurse, and she reached for her daddy's face the first time he held her. That "small" baby was 7 pounds, 12 ounces, 19 inches long, and was born totally naturally at 9:50pm. Our families were waiting in the waiting room and filed in two at a time to meet her (and bring us food and drinks because everyone was hungry!) By 2:00am I had eaten, showered, and been given two small stitches. We were home and making our way to bed with our little girl just five hours after she was born. I am so thankful for a healthy baby and a wonderful support system.

June

June 2, 2021

Tesereta and Israel: A Birth in Utah

I originally started out planning a hospital birth and told my OB that I wanted a natural birth. She seemed supportive, but a week before my due date she pushed me to schedule an induction. I really felt eerie and had the strongest feeling I needed to switch to a birth center. I'm a firm believer of following that gut feeling if it says something is wrong.

My husband and I were blessed to find a birth center that would take us in so late in pregnancy. Israel's expected due date was May 27th and it came and went. On May 31st at 2:00am, I started having mild contractions. They would start and then stop. The next evening my best friend, who was also my doula, came to meet me at a place where my husband was cleaning. She had me walk up and down stairs along with doing duck feet squats. Within a half hour, the contractions became more intense. Within an hour and a half, I was in active labor. Everything was happening so fast, and I was not prepared for how quickly everything was progressing. I had prepared for a long labor where things would be more spaced out because that is what I was taught happened with first time moms.

My best friend was so helpful. She knew the kind of birth I wanted. She respected it and did everything in her power to make it happen. From counter pressure, words of affirmation, rocking, and so much more, she kept me grounded. Around 8:30pm, we called the midwife to tell her that we felt I was in active labor. She didn't believe it at first because I was a first-time mom. She said to go home, take a bath, and that the contractions would possibly slow down.

We went back home and didn't make it to the tub because the contractions were coming back to back with hardly any break. The midwife said she would meet us at the birth center. We got there at around 9:30. I had to be hooked up to an IV to receive antibiotics for GBS, so I wasn't able to labor in the tub yet. When the midwife checked me, I was half a centimeter away from being fully dilated. There was a student midwife who was there and really helped me to manage the pain. She taught my support team other methods and techniques to help comfort me.

Around 10:00pm, I was able to get into the tub of water. By that time I was ready to push. I was really struggling with the fast labor and constant contractions. It was so exhausting.

I'm Polynesian. Polynesians really believe in our ancestors helping and supporting us. There came a point in the pushing process where my support team knew that they couldn't do much more for me and could only trust that I'd be able to accomplish birthing Israel naturally.

I remember closing my eyes and praying, "Please God help me. I'm so tired. Please send me my ancestors to support me." I remember a song from Samoa that talks about the strength of our Samoan women, and I instantly knew that my ancestors were there, watching over me and letting me know they were confident in me.

With that, my son came out with the next push. It truly was an empowering birth and an amazing first time experience.

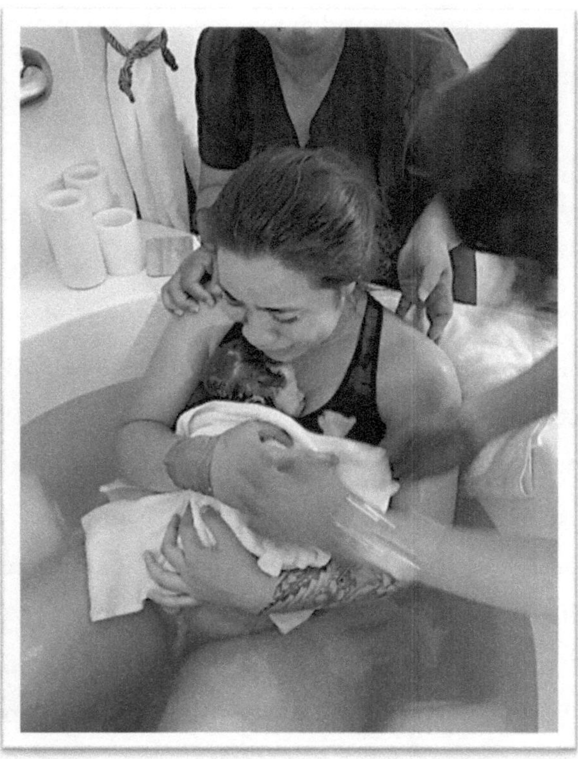

Natalie and Jones

I knew before I had even conceived my son that I wanted a homebirth. I had delivered my first child naturally at a birth center and loved the experience. I dreamt of a quiet, empowering water birth surrounded by my husband and close family. I dreamt about slipping into bed after delivering this child and introducing him to his older brother. I couldn't wait.

However, about 12 weeks into my pregnancy, I was diagnosed with both Gestational Diabetes and Complete Placenta Previa, which means my placenta was covering and blocking my cervix. With this condition, I was told there was no way to safely deliver a baby vaginally. If my placenta didn't move by the time I needed to deliver, I would need a planned Cesarean. My dreams of a natural home birth were crushed – and as I moved forward with planning for a C-Section, I worked to let go of the birth I had envisioned for so long. I simultaneously still held some small hope that my placenta would move before the birth.

Over the next months, I was put on pelvic rest. And no matter how hard I tried to keep my blood sugar low, those fasting numbers just kept rising. I was told that even if my placenta did move, now that I was on insulin to control my GDM, I would have to give birth in a hospital regardless. I felt out of control. Disconnected. I felt adrift. And I felt selfish and stupid for being so affected by all of this. Shouldn't my only concern be that my son is healthy? I should be thankful! But here I was, grieving my reality and letting go of the pregnancy and birth I had hoped for.

It was through this grief though that I was able to find acceptance, peace, and a newfound kindness towards myself. Of course, I want to do what is best for me and my son. Of course, I would choose the safest option. And don't even get me started on comparing my situation to other mamas who have it worse! But allowing myself to mourn the loss of my own expectations was perhaps the most healing part of this journey. And I can still feel empowered and birth my son in a way that felt honoring to us both.

I was able to find an OB who heard, listened, and saw me. An OB who let me talk about my fears, my wants, and desires for this birth without judgement. I found peace in being able to plan and advocate for the gentle cesarean that I desired. My son was born into a room full of individuals who were caring, kind, respectful, and joyful. There was no emergency and no panic. Just peace and excited anticipation followed by lots of skin to skin as they finished the surgery. It was not the birth I had initially dreamt of, but it was the birth I advocated for. It was the birth of my second sweet little boy, Jones.

June 10, 2021

Jodi and Everett

My estimated due date was May 30th. Braxton Hicks contractions began around 20 weeks and were pretty consistent and annoying. I constantly was reminding myself that this was my body preparing for birth. Around that same time, it became increasingly uncomfortable to recline at all. Even the slightest recline resulted in pretty intense contractions. My little man just didn't enjoy that position. With all of that, I was hoping that Everett would decide to be born around 39 weeks. I was feeling pretty large, uncomfortable, and very achy. Sleep was difficult. I had lots of insomnia. And, on top of that, I was experiencing prodromal labor off and on.

On May 15th, I began having some intense contractions. I was timing them and chatting with Patrice, my midwife, and we were pretty sure it was going to turn into something. My mom came to take the boys for the day. But the contractions fizzled out. I rested and had a low-key day.

May 26th also brought some excitement. The morning reminded me of the morning of Theron's birth. I slept great the night before. I was a little nauseated but also hungry and had good waves of contractions every 15-20 minutes that were more intense than I had felt yet. But they became less consistent and less intense as the day went on. By the next morning they were sporadic.

I didn't feel any consistent contractions again until June 5th. They lasted through the evening and we ended up with the whole midwife team here around 11:30pm. They stayed with me until about 2:30am when they got a call for another mother in labor. We all felt comfortable with them leaving because I was not progressing in labor symptoms, contractions were getting less intense again and baby stats were looking great. The next morning and afternoon, the sporadic and inconsistent contractions continued.

On Tuesday, June 8th, I woke with stronger contractions, but they still were not a regular pattern. His positioning felt different, and I made the drive to see Patrice one final time before baby arrived. I hadn't planned or desired to have a 41 week appointment. The next day was uneventful as far as my pregnancy goes. My oldest son, Michael, celebrated his 21st birthday that day and he and I talked throughout the day. He wanted to make sure he didn't have to share a birthday with his baby brother.

The morning of Thursday, June 10th, I sent this message to my midwife:

"I don't know what's happening. I have clusters of contractions that are 2 minutes apart for 5 or 6 cycles, then it stalls for 10-ish minutes, and then does it again. I had three cycles like this. They're definitely more intense though. I'm feeling super emotional and like I have no idea what I'm doing..."

After that I did the Miles Circuit with the stair lunges. Around 2:30pm I informed the midwife that I didn't need them to come. Nothing was really happening, and I was discouraged. I asked about considering a membrane sweep if we hadn't had any more consistent action soon. Early that evening I saw the chiropractor and had a great adjustment. He released a lot of tension in a ligament in my hip.

By 6:30pm I was having more regular contractions. My message to the midwife was:

"I don't feel like I can trust what's happening anymore because of all these false starts BUT just letting you know I've had 8-10 minute apart contractions for the past two hours. They are SUPER intense and low. I cannot walk or talk through them."

Within an hour the contractions were every 3-5 minutes and even more intense. We called the midwife, and the team headed our way! I was sure this was the real thing this time. Pete began to fill the pool.

With Theron's labor, getting in the pool provided almost instant relief and calmness. I did not experience that with this labor. I could not get comfortable and felt really agitated. I changed positions often. I got in and out of the pool multiple times and tried to find a more comfortable position. I tried lying in bed, I tried multiple positions in the pool, I tried standing and leaning over the bathroom counter while swaying back and forth. I could not find peace. I got back in the pool and labored more.

The contractions continued to intensify and get closer. Then, just after 11:00pm, one contraction came while I was leaning back in the pool and as it started, I knew I did not want to be in this position for the contraction. I started to get up to lean over the edge of the pool and experienced spontaneous rupture of membranes - my water broke! No more false starts. This was the real thing.

Pete called for the midwives who were downstairs. He let them know my water broke and they all came into the room. They checked the baby's heart tones every couple of minutes as I began to feel pushy. I stayed leaning over the edge of the tub and Pete sat down by me and took my hands. I felt surges of intense contractions that were pushing the baby down the birth canal for me. I was doing my best to just breathe and let my body work. The surges were coming right after another.

At one point, I felt him really moving down, and then when the surge paused, I thought I felt him move back up. In my head - and maybe even out loud - I said, "Oh no… I can't do this!" I thought I had so much work to do and that I was going to be pushing for a long time. At 11:32pm, we had a full crown, and I was able to reach down and feel his head. I could feel that he had a lot of hair and I started to talk to him. I remember saying that he was almost here and we were going to work together to do the rest.

During the surges I was letting out deep groans, but Barb and Pete were coaching me to have "blowing" breaths. They wanted me to pant and blow quick short breaths to stop myself from doing any actual pushing. We wanted my body to slow the process down and let him come on his own. This reduces the risk of tearing because the longer the baby takes to come out, the longer your tissues have to stretch. They had my best interests in mind, but it was so hard to just blow!

Patrice was providing tissue support from behind to really help my body and reduce the risk of tearing.

Just two minutes later, at 11:34pm his head was born… and then his arm came out immediately next! Baby rotated as needed.

At 11:35pm Everett Randall Sodini was born.

Instinctually, I reached down and grabbed him out of the water and brought him to my chest. Then I laid back in the pool and was given a towel to wrap him in. I began to soak in all of that moment and felt the massive surge of oxytocin. I felt so grateful, so alive, so primal and capable! I also noticed he was a BIG baby… but so was Theron, so I guessed he was about the same size. Somewhere around 11 pounds.

I stayed there in the birthing pool for a few minutes and thought I'd stay there to birth the placenta, but started to feel uncomfortable sitting. Since maneuvering with a baby attached to me is a bit complicated, we waited a bit longer - until the cord stopped pulsating - and decided to cut the cord before I moved. Midwife Kelsey clamped the cord and Pete cut it. Then we wrapped up Everett and handed him off to Pete (who snuck into the bathroom to see if he could get a weight with him and guess his size.)

I was able to get up and out of the tub easily and transferred to the bed where we had a bunch of blue pads down. I was given a smoothie and water and drank them down quickly. The midwives were checking Everett over - weighing, measuring, and assessing him. He was perfect. And weighed in at 12 pounds, 1 ounce, and was 22 inches long.

I was still sipping on my smoothie, and midwife Kelsey said I needed to try pushing a little more to get the placenta out. It had been about 45 minutes already. I didn't feel contractions and I was so tired and worn out. I just pushed when I could, and nothing was happening. The closer we got to an hour, the more discussion there was about needing to get this moving along. We discussed using an herbal tincture, but did not have what we needed on hand. Discussions of a hospital transfer were happening, and I began to feel a bit worried.

Apparently, the cut off for home birth regulations and the delivery of the placenta is 2 hours. So, at the one-hour mark, we got more serious. I did not want to go to the hospital. I didn't know what would happen with Everett or if I'd end up in surgery. I simply did not see transferring to the hospital as something that I could let be my reality.

I told Pete to grab the homeopathy book and look up "retained placenta". So he ran downstairs to grab it and came back up - he had found 3 remedies that were a possibility. We read about each and decided upon one. Sepia 30c - the description fit me best. So I took one dose every 15 minutes for 3 doses. That put us at the one hour and 40 minute mark. Then I decided I needed to pee, so I went to the bathroom and sat on the toilet. My mind started racing again about the logistics of a hospital transfer and I knew I did not want that. Finally, I was able to pee and then started to feel a contraction, so I pushed, and out came the placenta! Finally! Apparently, my full bladder could have made it difficult for it to come out.

I got help getting back to bed and got to hold Everett again and just soaked in all of the blessings and goodness I had just experienced.

Finally, the midwives had a chance to examine me to determine if any stitches were needed. We were all tired and it was after 2:00am at this point. Patrice determined that a couple stitches might be helpful for the healing process, but that they needed rest before moving ahead with that. So, they went downstairs to sleep in the living room and planned to come up in the morning. But those plans didn't last long. Around 3:00am, they got a call from another mother in labor, so they let me know they would be leaving and coming back as soon as they could.

Big brothers Fischer and Theron came in to meet Everett the next morning. We were so exhausted, but it was such a joy to see the boys so excited that Everett was finally here.

The midwives came back around 8:00am after the other mother's labor had stalled and they got some rest at her house. Patrice put in 3 stitches, and I was told to stay in bed with minimal activity for at least a week to properly heal. It's been a challenging recovery with a two-story home, but I can't say I'm not enjoying having breakfast in bed almost daily.

June 12, 2021

Alicia and Truitt: A Birth in Arizona

It was a warm Saturday morning when I was awakened by my water breaking while I was still in bed. I called my midwife and informed her of what happened and told her that I was not in labor yet. I was now on a clock to avoid having to go to the hospital because of midwifery license laws. I wanted to continue with my home birth plan. My husband and I decided to load up our two big kids and head to the park so I could walk around for a while and try to kickstart labor. After that didn't work, we headed home to meet with the midwife and get checked out. We also wanted some advice on how to get things moving.

We decided on belly lifts (ouch) and if that didn't work by 7:00pm I was going to drink a midwife's brew milkshake – castor oil, egg white and chocolate ice cream. I drank this at 7:45 and by 8:30 I was having consistent contractions. Around 10:15 I was on the toilet and having intense contractions. I was texting with my midwife, and she was getting ready to go to sleep. About 15 minutes later my contractions were back-to-back and not giving me time to relax. I told her to come on over.

She arrived at 11:05pm and started blowing up the birth pool with my husband. A few minutes into that I had a very intense contraction on the toilet. I felt down and was pretty sure I felt his head. I called out and said, "I think you should come in here, I'm pretty sure I feel his head!" This was at 11:25, only 20 minutes after my midwife arrived at my door. Chaos erupted, my midwife came in, felt his head, then instructed me to get off the toilet to which I replied, "I don't know how!"

My husband ran to grab my mom from the other room where she was laying down with my son. The midwife tasked my mom with collecting towels, and I made my way off the toilet. I took my position, standing up in the toilet room doorway, about to have my last contraction. I used gravity to effortlessly allow my third child and second son to enter the world.

Thankfully, my mom was able to grab a phone at the last second to record his birth. I reached down and brought him to my chest. He breathed his first breath as I caught mine, exasperated from all the adrenaline and oxytocin running through my veins. My sister and my daughter were just next door and made it to the room about ten seconds too late to see my son's birth. We made our way to bed and the midwife continued our checks for him and me. We took some time getting to know each other and nursed for the first time. He had a little more difficulty at the beginning than my other two babies did, but we figured it out together. He was born with a double knot in his cord;

apparently this is a rare phenomenon and thankfully we did not have any issues as a result.

He was a perfectly healthy, 9 pound, 22 inches long babe. He was my biggest and longest baby and my easiest birth. My daughter was overjoyed to be the one who got to cut his cord. My small room was full of love: my family, my mom, my sister and best friend held space with us while we got to know our newest addition into the early hours of the next day. I am so thankful for my midwives and home birth. It really allows the best environment for welcoming a child and for feeling safe and relaxed.

June 13, 2021

Nikole and Leilani

I woke up from a dead sleep at 1:30am with contractions. I didn't know for sure if this was the real deal yet, since I'd been having a lot of Braxton Hicks and still had seven days until my actual due date. I got out of bed, went into the kitchen, and grabbed the island as my contractions started to get stronger. They were already only a couple of minutes apart. I leaned into the counter to try and work through the waves. My mother was up sitting on the couch and asked, "Is it go time?"

I said I thought so, and that the contractions were in my lower back. I then grabbed my exercise ball, put it in the middle of the living room and started bouncing on it. I texted my midwife, Brea, my birth photographer, Carey, and my mother-in-law. I let them know I was having contractions. Carey and Brea asked how far apart my contractions were and suggested that I should start timing them. My mom went and woke my husband up and told him I was in labor. He jumped out of bed and started to fill the birthing tub while I bounced on my ball to help with contractions. At this point my contractions were getting longer and more painful. My midwife let me know that she was finishing up with a birth and would be on her way soon. She had texted Maddison, another midwife, to head over.

I continued to bounce on my ball and got a text from my photographer saying that my midwife was knocking on the door. My husband opened the door and said, "Umm, no one's out here." Five minutes later, Maddison got there and I felt such relief! She started to set up while telling me that she went to the wrong Nikole's house - we both laughed. At this point I moved my ball to the area where I was going to birth. After a few minutes of bouncing on the ball, Maddison helped me off the ball and into the birthing pool so I could try to relax my body. Right after that, Carey got there and immediately set her things up. My contractions were getting so hard to deal with that I don't even remember seeing Carey take pictures or film, she was like a secret ninja. Now my mother was walking around, my niece who was staying the night was up on the couch watching me, and my 4-year-old and 2-year-old were sleeping. It was about 2:30am and I tried to get out of the birthing pool because my contractions were killing me! Maddison grabbed my arms and in a soft spoken voice said, "If you get up, you will have to get out and go to your bed, you can't be half in and half out of the water."

I then said, "I think I'm going to poop!" I went to the side of the pool and my husband helped hold me up. I could feel her coming! Maddison checked and realized she was already coming. I put my hands near my vagina and I felt the top of her head. My heart got excited, but my body was in pain! At this point I remember letting out a couple of loud screams and my midwife told me to hold them in because it would help push her out. At 2:46am, Leilani Nikole made her way out and was placed on me. Then the front door opened and my oldest daughter and mother-in-law walked in. I was so overjoyed with emotion and was so happy that she was finally out. I didn't even notice that she was not crying or moving a ton. But then she started to make some grunting noises. I thought that was normal and I didn't think anything of it.

My midwife, Brea, got there and her and Maddison helped me out of the pool and onto the couch. I laid on the couch with my youngest daughter on my chest. I was so happy. I had my husband right next to me telling me he's so happy and that I did amazing. My midwives got my heating pad and placed it on Leilani. I still thought everything was fine. Brea then tells me they need to help get my placenta out and would push on my stomach. Not going to lie, that hurt almost as much as birth. We tried to get her to latch and see if she was hungry, but she didn't want to. I still think everything is fine. When they said Cody could cut the umbilical cord, I was happy! They then took Leilani and started to do something on the couch with her. Honestly, I didn't think anything of it and I assumed they were getting all of her information like her weight and height. I remember Brea holding her up and she was purple and limp. Then she said they needed to call 911 and we needed to go to the hospital.

My heart sank and I just cried while my husband said, "Of course, do what you need to do!" Within minutes, the fire department and EMS get there. I am literally naked on the couch, with my daughter on my chest. I felt like I was in Grey's Anatomy because all of these good-looking fire fighters come in. I made a joke to my husband "Never thought this many people would see me naked." My husband helps put my nightgown on and then my midwives help put my adult diaper on and I load up on the stretcher with Leilani in my arms and they put an oxygen machine on her to help her breath. I remember them loading us up into the ambulance and once we got in, I noticed that the oxygen was helping her and that her skin tone was starting to get pink. My heart was still sad because I couldn't help but think this was my fault, as I feel any mother would.

The guys in the ambulance were asking questions and all I could think was I didn't want to be in there and that this was not part of the plan. I remember just really only paying attention to my daughter on my chest and watching my husband driving right behind us. We finally got to the ER and the entire place was lined up waiting for us. I felt so weird and I didn't understand why so many people were there. My husband finally was next to me when I am being moved to a wheelchair and they put Leilani into a little mobile crib. One nurse asked us if we had her in the ambulance and I told them no, I had her at home in a birthing pool. She then looked at me with confusion and asked, "Are you sure? I then looked at her with a confused face and said, "Yes, I'm positive. She said, "Okay, someone must have mixed it up. They thought you gave birth in the ambulance." It then made sense why so many people were there waiting for us. They finally took us up to a room to have me checked out. Everything looked fine and they told me I could either get checked in or we could go up to the NICU where they had Leilani. I said I wanted to go to the NICU since nothing was wrong. The nurse wheeled me up into her room and she was already hooked up to oxygen, a heart monitor and a feeding tube was down her throat. My heart just broke because I didn't want to see her in any pain. But my husband and the nurses reassured me that this okay and it happened because she came so fast. It made me feel a little bit better, but until we were home, I wasn't going to feel that great.

For the next four days we would go back-and-forth from the hospital to the house. I am not going to lie, I always thought I was going to be able to give birth in my birth pool and have all my kids right there with me. I always imagined that once she was born, we would all be in the bed together looking at her, watching my midwives put her in the sling to weigh her, laying her flat on the bed to measure how long she was. Instead of doing all of that, our experience was a little bit different. We would FaceTime our kids so they could see their new sister. They put her on a scale to let us know that she was 8 pounds even and the nurses measured her and she was 20.8 inches long. Even though this was not in my birth plan, I am just so happy we had our amazing midwives who helped me deliver and made the call to move to the hospital. I am thankful for the nurses in the NICU who made Leilani's stay there more bearable.

My midwives and photographer were amazing and were always checking in on us. I am forever grateful for them! After our four-day stay, we finally got to go home and start our life as a family of six!

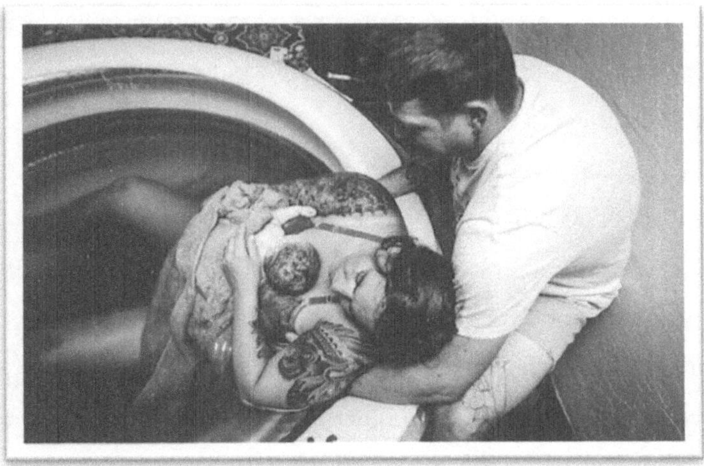

Photo by Carey Lauren
Carey Lauren Photos & Film

June 18, 2021

Andrea and Kirra

Early labor started on Thursday, June 17th. Contraction started waking me up around 2:00am. I contacted the midwife, and she said to rest as much as possible. At 8:00 the next morning, I had a bloody show. I did not want to eat or drink. I just felt crummy and it lasted all day. By 6:00pm I was only dilated to 3 centimeters. I felt like I should have been farther, so that was a disappointment to hear. My midwife said to take a bath and try to rest. I took a bath and while in the tub, my husband was giving me chicken, which tasted good until the nausea hit hard. Everything came up...

Contractions ramped up and our birth team started trickling in. My midwife showed up at 11:00pm and was checking on baby, who was doing great through the contractions. At midnight I was fully dilated and went into the pool. I started pushing and pushed from 2:00am- 4:00am. All the while I was throwing up every 15-20 minutes. Anything that went in came right back up. It was terrible. At one point while I was throwing up, I was throwing up so hard I had to mentally tell myself, "You can't breathe right now otherwise you're going to aspirate."

At 5:00am I was getting tired, so I got out of the tub and tried resting in bed. My water had not broken so the midwives broke it, which caused the contractions to get more intense. When they did this, they said I went from fully dilated down to 7 centimeters from swelling. There was talk about a hospital transfer, but we really wanted to avoid it, so we tried other things. We tried walking around outside but that did not last long so we got back into the tub. It was about 9:00am when we checked again, and I went down to 6cm… This whole time baby was stable with strong heart tones. We decided that we would transfer for maternal exhaustion and dehydration and get an epidural and fluids.

We got to the hospital around 11:00am on June 18. We got to the room and after going through all of the Covid protocol while still having contractions and nausea, I finally got anti-nausea meds which were a lifesaver! Thankfully, my home birth midwife was able to be there with us and we were able to have a nurse midwife from the hospital. I got the first epidural at 1:00pm and after an hour it hadn't worked and I ended up getting a second epidural. In between, my husband left and came back into the room to me getting the second which he had no idea was happening. They both hurt so goddamned bad, and I was black, blue, and purple afterwards. I don't ever plan to get another if I can help it.

The second epidural worked about eighty percent of the way and I was finally able to rest, so my home birth midwife left to get some food. I was able to eat, thank the lord, and was able to get some strength before I fell asleep. I was delirious and remember people coming to talk to us and thinking, "What an interesting dream - Oh, crap, that's the anesthesiologist. I should pay attention" and then fell asleep again. I slept until 6:00pm. When I woke up, I felt great and chatted with the nurse midwife. I started Pitocin after that and at 8:00 I was 8 centimeters dilated and at 10:00 I was fully dilated again. I started pushing again around 10:30pm and pushed for about an hour. Our daughter was born at 11:34pm on June 18, 2021.

The next morning, I was able to chat with my nurse midwife and she mentioned she was happy with how it all turned out, even with the barriers we had faced, and I agreed. She then informed me that I was minutes away from a C-section multiple times, which was what I was trying to avoid. Her overseeing medical doctor was stationed outside of our door after the first epidural and wanted to start Pitocin immediately, but she said no. Then, when Pitocin was started, he wanted to come in again to say C-section without even seeing what Pitocin would do. And he wanted to come in a third time at 8:00pm because he said, "There's no way she will be dilated again," yet to his amazement, we were progressing, and he finally stopped trying to force it.

Overall, we learned a lot with that experience, and I truly am very happy with how it turned out. Everyone comments about how it was so traumatic, but I don't feel that it was. It just wasn't what we had planned. I have things that I know I will change for the next birth... like taking anti-nausea meds right away!

June 20, 2021

Emily and Quinn

Around 9:30pm I woke up with what I would call my first contractions. I decided not to wake my husband up and actually liked the silence and solitude in the house. My goal was to let my husband sleep until midnight, but when I could no longer sit and rock through contractions and walking the hall stopped being manageable on my own, I woke him up. It was sometime around 11:30pm. He walked the hall with me, holding my hand and talking me through it all.

Around 1:30am is when I told him we needed to call people. My contractions were coming faster and faster and even talking was getting hard. We spent the next hour together, with him being my rock during contractions - letting me hold his arm and shoulders while I squatted down and back up. I squeezed him. When the contractions would let up, he would offer water and help me put my hands on the foot of the bed for a break. The second another contraction came, he would be right there for me to grab and squeeze while I squatted back. Finding a rhythm like this with him was so amazing. It was dependable and he was right there, holding space and making me feel safe enough to let go of my thinking mind and be deep in my birthing body. He would talk through each contraction, reading my affirmations and coming up with his own… even when I was so loud that I'm not sure if he could even hear himself say it!

Our midwife and doula got there around 2:30am. I barely knew they had come in other than the fact that I got to listen to the baby's heartbeat. That, along with hubby affirming everything, kept me so centered. Every time I heard her heartbeat it was like time stopped, pain stopped, and it was just me and her.

Around 3:00am my midwife suggested that I try to go to the bathroom and while sitting on the toilet I felt my body switch from contractions to pushing. I consciously just allowed my body to push when it was ready and didn't push extra or brace against it. After a bit my legs started to hurt from sitting, so we went back to the foot of the bed. I was on my hands and knees laying over the yoga ball. This was a great way to take a rest between pushes. By now my legs were exhausted and although I never felt like I couldn't do it, I was a little overwhelmed at how I was going to keep going when my legs were literally giving out. Again, my husband helped more than he will ever realize by saying, "You were made to do this, I know you've got this." I thought to myself, "If he believes in me so much, I must be able to do this".

I moved from the foot of our bed to the bathroom to be able to sit on the toilet and give my legs a break. Within what seemed like only a few more pushes I felt what is incredibly aptly called the ring of fire.

"She's coming," I said.

I had this new clarity about how I needed to think my way through this part and not let my body rush it. I moved from sitting on the toilet to my knees right in front with my yoga ball to lean on and husband to squeeze. I had laser focus on baby and silently talked to her about how this needed to be slow and how I really needed her to be patient. I breathed through each push trying to hold that burn instead of getting to the other side.

At 3:32am, Quinn Olive decided there was no more waiting and came to meet us. My midwife caught her and gently put her on the pillow between my legs. I told everyone I needed a minute and took time to breathe and savor the fact that I had done it!

June 28, 2021
Krista and Benaiah

I was lying in bed at 5:30am on a Sunday morning and woke up with a strange feeling in my abdomen. Since this was my first time being in labor, I wasn't sure what to expect and my baby's due date was still a few days away. I tried to sleep, since I knew I'd need energy, and wanted to ignore labor for as long as I could. But I was also keeping track of how long it was between contractions, and they were consistently coming every 10 minutes.

Around 7:00, I knew I must be in labor and couldn't sleep anymore. I texted my midwife and woke up my husband. Then immediately after telling him I was in labor, I got nauseous, ran to the bathroom and threw up. My husband jumped out of bed, came to the bathroom and started repeatedly asking, "What do we need to do?" I told him there was nothing to do right away since I was in early labor and it was going to take some time. I went about the morning getting ready for the day, cleaning the kitchen, and preparing a few things for birth and postpartum. The morning faded into the afternoon and friends brought over hamburgers for lunch. I tried to eat as much as I could while sitting on the birth ball, but I didn't have much of an appetite.

All afternoon my contractions were coming consistently and a little closer together as the day went on. Around 5:00pm it felt like the contractions were getting harder to cope with, so we decided to have our doula come over. She set up string lights in the bathroom and bedroom, put oil in the diffuser, and started vacuuming the house since we were managing the contractions fine without her. The contractions were manageable as long as my husband would push on my lower back to give counter pressure. He was so great the whole time, ready to apply counter pressure as soon as my next contraction started.

Day changed to night and things felt the same. We thought the contractions were closer together and getting more intense, so we had our midwife and assistant come around 10:30pm. They unpacked and around midnight the midwife suggested I lay down to sleep. I got all tucked in on my left side with a peanut ball between my legs and then threw up several times. In the early morning I did the Miles Circuit and labored on the toilet and birth ball.

Around 5:00am on Monday my contractions felt more intense, so we called my mom and I got into the birth pool. It felt nice in the pool and I decided to switch from listening to the hypnobabies tracks to my labor playlist which was a sweet moment. I tried different positions in the pool, but labor slowed down, so I got out. At this point we were all getting more serious about helping labor pick up. I tried many different tricks, but I still was not progressing much. Later that morning I was getting desperate, so I started bouncing hard on the ball trying to get my cervix to open up. Before 11:00am I remember surrendering to my labor and telling myself to stop fighting the contractions. I broke down crying on the birth ball, saying I just wanted to hold my baby.

Everyone on the team encouraged me and said to let my emotions out. After that I went back to laboring on the toilet and in the shower and the midwife, assistant, and doula decided to go get lunch. My husband and I rested while they were gone. Labor didn't pick up, so they all asked if I was alright with them going home to get some rest. I thought it'd be fine, and the midwife gave us several things to be on the lookout for.

During the afternoon I tried the Miles Circuit again, and slept when I could, waking up during contractions. Around 6:00pm I was watching a show on the birth ball and had several 5-7 minute long contractions. I'd get hot during and then cold between contractions. I called the midwife since the long contractions were unusual and she said we could go to the hospital to have the baby's heart monitored and that she'd be leaving right away. She also said to drink water with baking soda to break down the lactic acid which was probably what caused the long contractions. I got worried about the baby since I hadn't felt any movement but decided to stay home since the midwife was on her way.

At 8:18pm I was laboring on the toilet and my membranes ruptured. The amniotic fluid was a dark green. I knew there was meconium in the fluid, which meant the baby could be in distress. Labor really picked up and I could feel the baby's head so low. My body was pushing at the peaks of contractions. I felt like I shouldn't push yet because the midwife wasn't there and I wanted to give birth in the pool, not on my bedroom floor! I started panicking and hyperventilating, but my mom was right by my side helping me calm down and breathe deep and slowly. We called my doula. I tried to stop myself from pushing. After what seemed like forever (about 30 minutes), the midwife arrived, and my husband told her my water had broken. She noticed I was pushing and rushed around getting ready. Her assistant was driving separately and wasn't there yet, so our doula became her assistant.

By this time the water in the pool had cooled, but I was set on birthing in it. My husband and mom were boiling water and getting hot water from the bathtub. I was so ready to get in the pool and kept asking if it was ready. Finally, it was warm enough. I relaxed and let my body push. In the pool, I was sitting with my legs to the side, so I'd be ready to catch my baby. The midwife told me I could touch the baby's head and it felt squishy, not what I expected. She told me I was going through the ring of fire, and I thought to myself that it wasn't that bad. She had me pant to keep relaxed and reduce tearing and the head came out!

At 9:20pm I pushed again, and I caught the baby underwater. The cord was wrapped around the neck and torso, so the midwife held the baby still underwater and quickly unwrapped the cord. I brought the baby up to my chest and everything felt perfect. The baby was finally here! The baby had a little trouble breathing so I asked the midwife to use the nose aspirator to clean out his airways. The baby cried and I kissed my husband. We found out it was a boy! The placenta was taking a little while to detach, so I took a few herbs and then was able to gently pull it out on the toilet. He latched quickly and we got snuggled into bed for the first time as a family of three after about 40 hours of labor.

July

July 2, 2021

Audrey and Eden: A Birth in New York

In one word, my first pregnancy, labor and birth were…boring. I was low-risk in every way. I went into labor on my own at 41 weeks and 5 days and gave birth to my first baby after about 13 hours. "You'd be an excellent candidate for a homebirth," both doulas said during my postpartum care visits.

So here we were! About 7 months deep into a huge pandemic with hospitals placing restrictions on support for birthing people. Homebirth just made sense. I didn't want to have to worry about who would or could be with me during birth. I didn't want to worry about having birth plans change at the very last minute. And, after one unmedicated birth, I knew what I was capable of.

Fast forward 9 months of (boring!) pregnancy with a new birth team. We were ready. The birth pool was inflated. The homebirth kit was acquired. The plan for our 2 year-old was set. Then my husband got incredibly sick when I was 40 weeks and 3 days. I was working from home and was frantic – I called his doctor and tried to get him scheduled for a Covid test, but he could barely move, eat or drink. I dreaded the idea of doing this without him or, worse yet, asking my birth team to enter my home that may be Covid positive. I worried about if I needed a transfer to the hospital and had to be in a "neutral" area without my husband. We had already had Covid earlier in the year, and his symptoms this time seemed different, but we still worried.

The next day I had off from work for the 4th of July weekend. My husband slept in our guest room, and I remember waking up on and off throughout the night. I woke up with my toddler at 6:00am and soon realized that I had been waking up because I was having sporadic contractions. I woke up my husband and told him I was pretty sure today was the day. He was feeling a bit better, thankfully, but was still weak from not eating or drinking much the day before. My mom, who was staying for the birth, brought over muffins, and my toddler and I played in the birthing pool (not filled) until it was time for my dad to come get him.

For the next few hours my husband handled texting our birth team. I just focused on the surges. I wasn't even timing them, really, just figuring out where I was the most comfortable. My doula/midwife assistant appeared around 8:45 and the midwife soon after. I was fully engulfed in the contraction fog and didn't have a sense of time. I was just riding the waves.

I really tried listening to my body and not worrying about what was going on around me. I was in a safe space, and I focused on that. I labored in the living room, on the floor, on the couch, and in the bathroom. Our doula suggested moving to my bed and I was in a side-lying position when I transitioned. She said the pool was ready and I was welcome to move whenever I wanted. Contractions were getting really rough. I remember, in a brief moment of stillness, just blurting out that it felt like my hips and pelvic bones were being crushed. In reality, they were making space and that meant progress. I got in the pool and felt my whole body relax.

I had voiced wanting to catch my baby when the time came, so my doula encouraged me to explore with my hands during the contractions. Feeling my baby's head start to emerge and how instantly my body just opened to allow her passage was absolutely shocking. Was it supposed to happen this quickly? Am I going to tear horribly? So, I stopped pushing. My husband was wiping me with a continuous stream of cool washcloths. It was such a welcome contrast to the other sensations happening in the rest of my body.

After what felt like an eternity, another contraction gave me the strength to push until her head was out. I could feel her slick, slightly mushy skull and parts of her face, but I kept my eyes closed. The relief when the rest of her body emerged and we lifted her onto my chest was just immense. At around 10:46am on July 2nd, Eden was born into my hands, surrounded by an incredible birth team and family.

July 4, 2021

Anais and Emilia: A Birth in Spain

My first delivery was traumatic. It was very intervened. I arrived at the hospital at 7 centimeters dilated, they gave me an epidural and then they artificially broke my waters without my consent. The epidural left me useless from the waist down, I stopped feeling absolutely everything. After seven hours, obligatory lithotomy position, directed pushing in apnea, an episiotomy and forceps, my 4,200 Kg (9 pounds) and 54 cm (21 inches) baby, was finally with me.

Postpartum was hell. I went through pelvic floor rehabilitation for rectocele and hemorrhoids. I had episiotomy scar tissue treatment due to adhesions. It took me a year to feel like myself again.

I often wondered about my birth. I wondered what would have happened in my birth without an epidural, if everything had gone wrong because of the size of my baby, why they didn't ask for my consent, why I wrote a birth plan that no one read, if the hospital had an equal birth protocol for all women, if my body failed at what it is supposed to be designed for...

My second pregnancy I decided to follow it up with a different Ob/Gyn and hire the One to One team (a birth center) at HM Nuevo Belén, a different hospital. I tried not to feel that childbirth is a kind of a disease, but rather a normal physiological process. It was the best decision I made.

I was diagnosed with gestational diabetes and it broke me down to think that my baby would be even bigger than her older brother. I read Lily Nichols, Midwife on the Wave (Comadrona en la Ola, a great Spanish midwife), Glucose Goddess and everything felt okay. I did AIPAP (pelvic training method in the pool) and bought the Get Mom Strong pregnancy exercise program. All went phenomenal and my baby was growing perfectly.

I was first monitored with my midwife from One to One at week 37. Everything looked good. We talked at length about my first birth and the whole intervention package that I received. It was therapeutic to talk about what I had been through. At week 38, I went to be monitored with the father and brought my 4-page birth plan. It included newborn treatment and what to do in case of a caesarean or perinatal death. We talked about it, we changed a couple of things, and my midwife explained to me that outside the birth center, hospital protocols would have to be followed. We decided to condense the plan into a single page and print it on a bright colored paper, so it wouldn't get lost in the wastebasket.

Sunday morning I was 39 weeks. I was woken up by what I would consider to be Braxton Hicks contractions, but they were painless. I didn't say anything to the father, he was sleeping peacefully. The contractions continued and started to hurt, like a severe period. Everything was fine. He woke up and the waves continued. I warned the father that he would not be able to go biking, that it may be a false alarm, but that I preferred not to take the risk. I started to informally count the frequency of the contractions - they seemed to appear every 10 minutes. We got up and had a typical breakfast since the diagnosis of GD: two eggs, avocado, goat cheese and cherry tomatoes. I include a slice of bread in case I would not be able to eat for a long time. I needed at least a few carbohydrates as gasoline to hold on. I also made myself a cup of milk and cocoa.

The contractions were now every five minutes, and we called the midwife. I think it was 11:00am. I told her that I was tolerating labor well with the birth ball and with other techniques that we learned in the course Childbirth and Movement of Physiospecialists. I took a shower, and I began to feel that it was a false alarm because the pain disappeared with the warm water. The father was outside asking what songs were supposed to be on the labor playlist that we hadn't made yet.

I got dressed and my sister arrived to stay with our oldest. The contractions were every two and a half minutes, maybe less, I finally felt like it was time to go to the hospital. We called the midwife to warn her. We asked for a taxi. Suddenly, I felt a contraction that bends my legs, it was the first one that was really excruciating. It's noon. I screamed and hit the bathroom door with my right fist, I couldn't stand up. I looked at the bed and thought about going to the bedroom. I can't because I feel an absurd desire to poop. We called the midwife, and she stayed on the phone. I went to the toilet and pushed. Some poop came out, but it was not really the urge to go to the bathroom that I felt. This was something else.

I got into the shower and immediately went on all fours. I felt like pushing some more. I screamed with everything that I had. I felt like I couldn't. The pressure was indescribable. I started to feel heat. No, not heat, I felt as if my legs were separated from my body with a flamethrower.

"I can't, I can't, I can't." I thought.

The midwife was on the phone, the father was by my side. The head came out and the relief was as indescribable as the pain I felt seconds before. I breathed in and out calmly while I waited for the next contraction. The father held her head. In the next contraction, I didn't even have to push, my uterus did all the work. The body came out completely. The father put her on my chest, the cord was short, it didn't have loops around the neck, but it did around one of her arms. She cried and was pink like a shrimp. I was so full of oxytocin. I couldn't believe it.

It was 12:15 p.m. on Sunday, July 4, 2021.

My midwife arrived 10 minutes later, straight from home. She had none of her equipment. I told her I felt like pushing. I delivered the placenta in two pushes, and we took it to the hospital in a plastic bag, still attached to the baby, in my midwife's car.

At the hospital, the gynecologist on duty sutured a second degree tear. The pediatrician saw my baby, the father cut the cord, and my midwife made an impression of the placenta. We went upstairs and the baby latched onto my chest. I was still in my cloud of oxytocin. Still unable to believe what happened. I got what I had dreamed of; that healing birth, that natural, ancestral physiological process, my empowered and capable body.

I am eternally grateful to those who made it possible. My team, Dr. Suárez (my ob-gyn), the wonderful One to One (the birth center), my midwife, my pelvic floor physio, the father of my children, my children and my family.

I feel complete.

To everyone reading, I wish you all the pregnancy and birth of your dreams. Because we can. It's imprinted in our DNA.

July 17, 2021

Jessica and Emma Grace

I had been having contractions on and off all week. I was over 41 weeks at this point, so I was starting to feel a little anxious. I knew I needed to deliver my baby girl this week or I would lose my chance to have her at home. I was cooking dinner and realized that I had been having contractions 5-8 minutes apart, very consistently. I was no longer able to mindlessly keep working. I had to stop and breathe through each surge. It felt like a switch had flipped – I was honestly in denial! I thought there was no way I could be in labor. I waited on contacting my midwife and tried all the tricks to "stop" my contractions to see if it was really labor. I called my midwife around 7:45 to let her know I was pretty sure this was it. It was my first baby, so I was feeling the sensations of labor for the first time.

By 10:00pm I was feeling pretty tired and decided to see if I could get some rest but lying down in bed was far from comfortable at this point. Surges were getting stronger, and I couldn't sleep through them.

I ended up walking outside for a bit and moving around the house - from the couch, to the bath, to the bed and all over again and again just trying to get comfortable. I called my midwife around 12:30am with a bit of weariness, letting her know I couldn't sleep and wasn't sure what to do. She encouraged me and gave me some pointers on how to get some rest. The emotional support alone was just what I needed. I was able to get comfy on the couch and rest through the night. I highly encouraged my husband to get some rest. I knew I needed him well rested for what was coming!

The next day was Friday, and I had some breakfast in the morning and then rested around the house. Debbie, my midwife, came over around 11:00am to take vitals and check on me. She brought so much peace and calm with her and let Jordan and I have the house to ourselves while I slowly let baby work her way out, hour by hour. She stayed close by at a coffee shop to come and check in when needed. By 3:00pm, she knew active labor had begun and stayed with us at this point. My mom and sister came over around 4:30 and helped get my husband some dinner. They jumped in to support me when needed and gave Jordan some breaks.

Around 7:00pm I was beginning to really feel strong urges and got into the birth pool around 7:30. Debbie's birth assistant arrived at this time as well. Being in the water took so much pressure off my back and belly, it was honestly so relaxing. My sister has a video of me in the pool saying, "I feel like I could take a nap." I began to feel like my body was pushing for me, like I couldn't help it. After about an hour or so in the tub, Debbie gently suggested that I try laboring over the toilet to let gravity help us. It was on the toilet that I reached down and could feel her head so close. It was encouraging to me, but I was so very tired. I was over 24 hours into labor at this point.

After laboring for about 45 minutes on the toilet, Debbie asked me what sounded good to me. I asked to lie on the bed, which was not the original plan, but it was what sounded good in the moment. They dimmed the lights to nearly dark, had cool cloths for my head and warm compresses for my perineum. With the room totally silent, I slept in between every contraction, in the comfort of my own bed. It was amazing. I had support from Jordan by my side. Sue, the birth assistant, held my leg when I was too weak to hold it myself. My mom and sister were the best cheerleaders.

Emma Grace Gentes was born at 12:48am on July 17th. They put her on me immediately and it was the greatest feeling ever, knowing what my baby girl and I had just accomplished. She latched to breastfeed like a champ and Debbie gently assisted while I delivered my placenta. We spent an hour in our room, just Jordan, Emma and I, in pure peace and bliss while my birth team cleaned up the rest of the house and made me some food.

It was soon after that Emma was sound asleep in my husband's arms while I got cleaned up and ready for bed. Debbie showed me the placenta which had to be one of the most amazing and fascinating things I have seen. I was so grateful she took the time to do that. It was around 3:00am when my little family was tucked into bed, Emma between us, ready for uninterrupted sleep to begin our recovery. Home birth is such a special gift that I hope every family can experience if they wish.

July 20, 2021

Emily and Ella Jane

My labor started on July 19th. I lost my mucus plug and had some bloody show and inconsistent contractions that evening. I went to sleep and woke up at 1:00am to stronger contractions that I couldn't sleep through, so I got up and told my husband I didn't think he'd be going to work that day.

We sat on the couch watching the Twilight saga on Netflix. At 3:15am my water broke. I called my midwife and doula to let them know, and they both recommended that I try and go back to sleep until things picked up. When I woke up that morning, my contractions were 5-7 minutes apart. I tried to go about my day as normally as possible. I did a lot of walking around in the house, sat on my birth ball, and watched tv while my husband took a nap because he had been working nights. By afternoon my contractions had stalled and spaced out anywhere from 10-20 minutes in between. My midwife asked me to come into the office to be checked since my water had broken.

I joked in the car on the way there how ironic it was because one reason I planned a homebirth was to not have to be in a car during active labor and my midwife's office was an hour away. Once I got to the office I was still smiling and joking around and my midwife checked me and told me, "You get the gold star of gold stars! You're 8 centimeters dilated. We're going to your house right now to have a baby!

By the time we got home at 6:00pm, my contractions were consistent. We weren't sure we'd have enough time to set up the birthing pool, so we decided not to. I must have been laboring for a while with no noticeable changes so my midwife had me walk the stairs and checked me again. I was still only 8 centimeters. She broke my second water bag and things got intense quickly. I pushed for about an hour and half total. Mostly in a side lying position and then I switched to hands and knees near the very end.

When her head came out I looked down and said, "Oh my god, there's a head!" My midwife told me with the next contraction my baby would be here. I could feel her turning her body working with me to be born, and then with the last push she was out! I was immediately able to sit back on my legs and pick her up and bring her to my chest. I have never felt such overwhelming joy and relief and love.

I never felt any pain until I started pushing. It was intense, but not painful until that point. Even though I didn't get the water birth I wanted, I still got a beautiful natural birth experience. Giving birth was the hardest, most intense thing I have ever done, but it was also joyful, transformative, and incredibly empowering. I still can't believe I did it.

July 29, 2021

Rosann and Izabelle and Avigail: A Twin Home Birth

I found out at 12 weeks pregnant that we were having twins. It was only two days after meeting with our midwife for the first time. The doctor told us we would have to have a c-section and that because I was pregnant with twins, it classified as a high risk pregnancy. My midwife disagreed and we decided we would go ahead with the home birth as planned. Fast forward to 39 weeks and 5 days. I was at the library with my husband and two older girls in the morning and felt some fairly strong contractions. I told my midwife about it but told her I wasn't concerned, and I'd call if it changed.

When dinner time came that night, my husband was at work and my parents came from over an hour away in case something changed while he was gone. Things hadn't changed and I sent my parents home around 7:30. Frustrated and wanting to meet my twins, I took a bath and tried to relax, then I went to bed around 9:00pm.

I woke around 12:15 with a very strong contraction and then woke my husband. I laid there and waited for another and knew it was time. I called my mom the midwife mid-contraction and was already to the point of barely being able to talk. She assured me she was on her way and that we were going to have babies that night.

I got out of bed and the contractions were very strong and coming every few minutes. I swayed and turned music on. My husband got things ready and our midwife showed up around 1:05am. Her assistant and my mom, both an hour away, were rushing to make it on time. My midwife quickly got her supplies out and prepared my floor and the bed. She helped me breathe through the contractions as my husband was making sure everything else that we needed was ready. I got in the shower for about five minutes and knew things had changed and I quickly got out and back to the bedroom.

I tried leaning over my bed but didn't feel comfortable and instead got on the floor on my knees and leaned into our gliding rocking chair. My midwife let me know that I could push at any time when I was ready.

And so I did.

I pushed and my water broke and then with the next contraction I pushed again, and her head was out. With one more push, at 2:04am my 5 pound 14 ounce Izabelle entered the world screaming. My husband grabbed her and handed her to me through my legs and I held her.

After Baby A was born, I got on the bed so my midwife could check the position of Baby B. She couldn't quite tell but told me that once my water broke she would be able to tell. Shortly after saying that, my water broke. While my husband went to get more towels, I pushed again and my sweet Avigail entered the world just as quiet as can be with big eyes just taking it all in. She was born at 2:19am and weighed 7 pounds 1 ounce.

The big sisters heard the cries and shortly after they joined us to meet their new twin sisters. My mom and the midwife's assistant made it shortly after the birth.

It was the most amazing and empowering experience of my life!

August

August 1, 2021

Chelsey and Sawyer

They say that each baby is supposed to come earlier than the last. My second and third babies were both born at 39 and a half weeks, so I thought for sure that my fourth would come at or before that. Week 39 rolled around, and I was looking for all the signs that labor might be starting. That week came and went. I was so surprised by this because I was sure our little one would have arrived by now. Then, week 40 came and almost went.

The day before 41 weeks, I woke up and started having contractions. They were very mild at first, but soon became stronger throughout the day. I kept telling my family it wasn't the real deal because these contractions were so irregular. They were about 40 seconds to a minute long, but they didn't come regularly at all. One would come, then the next wave would come in 20 minutes, and the following in 9 minutes, and the next in 5 minutes, another in 11 minutes. After a whole day of this I was exhausted.

We were at my mother-in-law's house for most of the day. I kept debating, "Do we want to leave and go to the hospital?" I wasn't ready yet and I think I knew that, but the exhaustion was setting in, so I called my midwife. My sweet midwife encouraged me, she analyzed everything I told her, and she said in her experience I would go into labor within a day or two. My husband and I packed our children and drove a short 15-minute drive home.

My body was tired, so I decided to get into a nice warm bath when we got back to the house. As I was in the bathtub, I started to notice that my contractions seemed to become more regular. I started timing them and sure enough they were 9 minutes apart. After getting out of the tub I tried to take a quick nap, but they quickly became 7 minutes apart and then 6. We headed to the midwife after my mother and father-in-law arrived at our house to watch our 3 boys. When we arrived, I was able to get right into the jetted whirlpool tub. I highly recommend this for natural pain relief! Being inside the warm water was very soothing to me. My husband lovingly snapped pictures as I breathed through each wave, and he talked with me next to the tub.

I spent almost 2.5 hours in that tub before I decided to get out. When I stood up, I immediately knew this baby would be coming soon. My legs trembled beneath me as I made my way over to the bed. I told my midwife that my last two babies came forcefully after the bag of water broke and she asked me if I wanted her to break my water for me. I gave her permission to do so. I was relieved when they said my waters were clear and my 41-weeker had not passed any meconium in the womb.

I laid on my back in the bed for a contraction or two. This baby didn't feel like it was going to fly out. I turned around on all fours and I felt the baby descending. Instinctively, I got into a squat on top of the bed and pulled my right leg up to the head rest. Within a minute, my sweet baby boy came earthside. He had bright blue eyes and very light and thin blonde hair. Almost immediately he latched to my breast. My fourth son, Sawyer Marshall, was born on August 1st, only 3 hours after arriving at the hospital. It was 2:00am and he was 9 pounds 13 ounces and 21.75 inches long.

August 3, 2021

Chelsea and Henry

By the third trimester, slightly peeing my pants had become the norm. So, on August 2nd when I came out of the shower and noticed a small gush of water splat on the floor, I chalked it up to another fun pregnancy moment! I spent the day grocery shopping and running errands. As the day progressed, I felt more and more drained. At 2:00am that night I woke up in a puddle and decided to get checked out. Two uterine fluid swabs later I was told I wasn't going back home and that my baby would be arriving soon. I cried. I wasn't ready! I still had 2 weeks! We didn't install the car seat! Did I even shave my legs?

I was induced at 5:00am and had no idea what to expect. I wanted to give birth as naturally as possible without an epidural. The first few hours the contractions were mild, and I thought, "I totally got this!" The summer Olympics were on TV, so I happily rode the contraction waves and chatted to the nurses about the Olympics as they came in and out. By noon the contractions had become more intense and severe back pain started kicking in. By 3:00pm the contractions were unbearable. I remember thinking it was the most painful feeling I'd ever experienced. I shed a few tears to my partner and decided I wanted an epidural after all. The nurses let me know that the anesthesia team was busy, but I was next in line!

The nurses gave me some morphine, which for a short time got me through the pain and allowed me to eat a coffee crisp chocolate bar that I had been craving. Then all of a sudden, I had to poop. The nurses seemed concerned and warned me not to push too hard. I remember thinking how silly that was, and I reassured them I definitely just had to use the bathroom. By the time I waddled to the toilet, my body had started doing something strange. Instead of the normal painful contractions, my entire body felt like it was uncontrollably tensing up. I was convinced there was something wrong and kept asking the nurses if this was normal. Was I ok? Was the baby ok? What was happening to my body?

A nurse quickly checked my cervix and yelled, "That's the baby's head, get the doctor!" It all came together at that moment. I realized my incredible body was doing the work and guiding me through the process of having my baby! I grabbed the nurse's arm.

"What about the epidural?" I begged.

"They won't make it in time, you can do this, your baby is coming!"

The doctor casually walked in with a big smile. At this point, I knew this was the home stretch. I pushed when they told me to push, took a few seconds to breathe when my body let me, and then pushed again. I can only describe the experience of birthing your baby as completely surreal. I was physically there but my mind was somewhere else - connected to the millions of other women in the universe who had gone through the same thing. At 5:31pm on August 3rd, my partner cut the umbilical cord and they handed me my goopy little wrinkly baby boy, Henry.

August 3, 2021

Candace and Magnolia: A Birth in Honolulu, Hawaii

Growing up, my mom always talked to me about birth, because I knew I wanted to have lots of kids. My mom had all three of us naturally and always said to me "It may be the worst pain that you will ever feel, but it will all be gone as soon as you hold that baby in your arms." Oh, how right she was! Magnolia came into the world on August 3rd at 2:36pm weighing 6 pounds 14 ounces. Everyone was shocked how big she was, because she was five weeks early...

On Tuesday morning, I got up to send my Air Force husband off to work at 4:00am and did my normal routine before work (which typically consisted of a nap at this point). I got up, ate some breakfast, and went to work. I had decided to not work this school year, but it was the first day of school and I was helping with evaluations. Around 8:30am, we did a bathroom break for the kids. I took one as well. When I came out I took a few steps and thought "Man, I just peed on myself." The next step I realized it was not pee! I told Kristy to get Kirsten (one of my best friends) and I went back into the bathroom. When Kirsten got there, she confirmed what I was thinking - that my water had broke. I was hysterical over the fact that I did not even have a bag packed at home for the hospital yet. She told me to call my husband while she went to get our principal.

I called Ben and there was no answer. I just knew he was on the flight line delivering munitions to the jets. I called Amanda, another Air Force spouse, and she told me she would call her husband to get Ben. I asked her to please come and get me and take me to the hospital. She took me to the hospital and stayed with me for about an hour until Ben got there.

In triage, I was feeling no contractions. They said I was having some based on the belly monitor, and I focused really hard to see what they felt like. During this time, the midwife on duty came in and did a fluid test to confirm that it was my water. She also did my GBS test since I was not 36 weeks yet and had not had one done. No cervical check was done due to my water being broken, and I did not want one anyways. They were talking to me a lot about taking antibiotics since I would not have the GBS results for a few days. They also talked about me taking a steroid shot to help the baby's lungs develop and what the timeline looked like before interventions would be recommended.

I was extremely overwhelmed. I had a birth plan, but it was at home on my computer. My amazing midwife continued to assure me that they would do whatever I wanted. At this point, it was around 11:00am. Ben and I had made a list of all the things he needed to get at home, and Amanda was going to meet him there to help. I was then moved out of triage into a delivery room.

Ben went with me to the delivery room, and then he headed home. My nurse was great the entire time during labor. The first thing she did was tell me that as long as she was the only one in the room, I did not have to wear my mask. She got my IV started with the antibiotics for unknown GBS results and had another nurse come do my COVID test. They hooked me up to the fetal monitor and gave me a birth ball, but I found that it was not very comfortable because I felt like I was sitting on my baby's head. I decided to stand since gravity is your best friend in labor. As I was rocking, my contractions started picking up. Around 1:00pm, Ben got back to the hospital and labor kicked in full force.

My nurse unhooked me from everything so I could move freely, and I chose to go to the bathroom to labor on the toilet. At this moment, I told Ben, "If I am only like 4 centimeters dilated, I do not know if I can do this!" He responded with, "You are not getting an epidural." (This was part of our birth prep. He knew his role!) I asked Ben to bring me my water bottle, because I felt really thirsty. Every time a contraction would come, I would stand up and rock back and forth while my arms were resting on a shelf above me. Then I would sit back down once it passed. I was starting to feel sick to my stomach and like I needed to poop. I felt like I couldn't catch my breath because the surges kept coming.

At 2:10pm I told Ben that he needed to get someone because I wanted to be checked. I just knew she was coming now! They checked me and told me to push or do whatever my body was telling me to do. No coached pushing. I wanted a cold rag on my face and my water between pushes.

The only time they gave me advice was to breathe and let her head sit for a moment when my cervix was stretched. A few pushes later, Magnolia was earthside! She was immediately placed on my chest. A male nurse was standing beside me checking on her for her breathing, since she was a preemie. Ben and I were so excited and overjoyed. Honestly, I do not remember the pain of having her because each surge was a moment closer to meeting our baby girl. I would have a natural birth 10,000 more times and ride those waves into this beautiful moment. Thank you, mom, for all the encouragement as a kid. And thank you to my husband for being right by my side through it all.

August 4, 2021

Carmen and Payson: A Birth in Arizona

On Sunday, July 25th, I woke up around 6:00am having contractions. I kept track of them, but nothing was consistent enough to send me to the hospital. After several hours they died down and then stopped altogether. They came and went sporadically for the next week and a half. The next Wednesday, August 4th, I woke up with contractions again and decided to try taking a shower to see if that would make them stop. It was the second day of school, so I sent my husband to take our oldest to the bus stop, but warned him to come back quickly.

He wasn't convinced it was real this time and took his time getting home. By the time he got home I could hardly walk or talk. We waited for a friend to pick up our youngest, and as soon as she was gone, we left the house. On the way to the hospital, which is about 15 minutes away, I mentioned that I'd been thinking about having this baby without an epidural, which I had never done before.

We arrived at the hospital around 9:00am and were taken to a room right away. My midwife arrived just after us. Baby boy had been sunny side up for weeks and we tried to turn him by doing rebozo techniques. My contractions were long and hard. My midwife said, "Did you feel that? He turned. These are baby flipping contractions!"

My water broke pretty dramatically after that and I began to really feel the need to push, but I couldn't push on my back. I didn't have the stamina or strength. I asked if I could get on my hands and knees and my midwife told me I could do whatever I needed. I turned over and only pushed a few times before my sweet baby boy was born at 10:21am No time for an epidural anyway! I have never been so tired and so proud.

Kennan and Knox

I'd been having early labor signs for a week and a half, and was getting frustrated that they weren't going anywhere. I'd have Braxton Hicks for 3 or 4 hours at a time each day, but they'd always fizzle out. On Thursday, July 29th, I had my first cervical check and was 1 centimeter dilated and 70% effaced. My cervix was already forward and soft. My body was doing what it was supposed to. I lost my mucus plug on Saturday, July 31st and had cramps most of the day on Sunday. But nothing else happened.

I had a non-stress test scheduled for 1:30 on Wednesday, August 4th. The test went great. Baby was healthy and responding well. It picked up good heart rate accelerations and it was a good indication that he would handle labor well. My midwife checked my cervix again. I was 2 centimeters and about 80% effaced. Not a huge change from the week before, but progress. During the check, she felt that the baby's head was tucked slightly and not completely anterior like we would ideally hope for. I went home with plans to do the miles circuit and forward leaning inversions to hopefully get his head in a better position.

Almost immediately after the cervical check, I began having menstrual type cramps that were pretty strong. Something about these cramps felt different. I still can't put my finger on why they felt different, or how, but they did. We got home and I started the miles circuit. I talked to my mom and sister on the phone, watched Netflix, and the cramps continued. By 6:00pm they seemed to come and go in a rhythmic fashion. Every 10 minutes or so a cramp would come on. They were low, just like a bad period cramp. I let my midwife know.

At 9:00pm I went to the bathroom and on the tissue was bloody show. I texted the midwife and her suggestion was to get in bed and rest. I asked my husband, Elisha, to pack his bag just in case it was time. This took about an hour and by then, my contractions were four and a half minutes apart and lasted about 45 seconds. They had become much stronger, but didn't feel anything like the Braxton Hicks I'd experienced last week. They stayed mostly in my pelvis. Low and consuming. I had to sway back and forth to ease discomfort. My midwife let me know she was going to rest and get ready for me to let her know when my demeanor had shifted and my contractions were four minutes apart, lasting at least a minute, for at least an hour.

The next few hours were spent working through contractions. Elisha supported me and we used our techniques we'd been practicing. Breathing, low sounds, swaying, the birth ball, forward inversions. What I remember most from this time is the pain in my back. The contractions didn't feel anything like contractions, but rather my pelvis becoming engulfed in heat. At this point they were 4 minutes apart and lasted between 55 seconds and 80 seconds, so we called the midwife. It was 12:40am. She said to meet us at the birth center in an hour and a half. I called her back 20 minutes later because I wasn't feeling any tightening in my belly, just the pain in my pelvis and I wanted to ask her opinion. She recommended more forward leaning positions and actually told us to wait a little bit longer based on how I was talking. I was coping well with contractions, but the thought started to creep in - "I don't know how long I can do this."

The next hour and a half was intense. I had to empty my bladder multiple times and this pain was the worst. Having to sit down and stand back up and walk during a surge was not easy, even with my breathing techniques to help me. The majority of this time was spent with me in child's pose on the floor in our living room with Elisha applying counter pressure during every contraction. Around 2:30, we called the midwife again and made plans to meet at the center at 3:45. This last hour at home was hard. My demeanor had certainly shifted, and I was in labor land. I don't remember a lot of what I was thinking other than what I said earlier - my body was doing what it was supposed to. There was that creeping thought in the back of my head though. "What if we get there and I'm only 4 centimeters dilated. I'm not going to be able to do this much longer."

At 3:15, we started packing up to head to the center. It was a 20 minute drive. I had two surges on the stairs on the way down to the car and these were hard to get through. I was no longer in my space or comfortable. When I was standing, my back pain was overwhelming. When I was tilted over it subsided, but there was no way to lean over on the stairs. Or in the car for that matter. The car ride was the worst. No comfort at all. I just had to get through it. The doubt in the back of my mind was strongest in the car. "If I'm not progressing, I'm going to have to go to the hospital."

We arrived at the center and our birth videographer was close behind us. It took me several minutes to get inside. The midwife greeted us, and I had to lean over the bed so I could get the pain off my back. She asked my permission to check my cervix after we got somewhat settled (Elisha parked the car and brought in the bags). I told her, "Yes, but I'm scared. What if I'm not far along?" She reassured me that based on the timing of the surges and my demeanor that she was sure I was making progress. She checked my cervix and to my surprise I was 7 centimeters dilated! Seven! I had renewed energy. Renewed faith in my body. I could do this. I kept thinking "open" and "soft" through my surges. I didn't fight them. I leaned into them and knew that they were doing hard, good work. I needed to empty my bladder and had several surges facing backwards on the toilet. This wasn't my favorite position. We moved next to the shower. Elisha held my hand as I sat on a birth ball and he held the shower head on my lower back. I was here for maybe 45 minutes. I was in a really good headspace here. I was trusting my body. The surges were stronger than they had been, but I was handling them better. Elisha even asked if they had stopped coming, he couldn't quite tell when I would get one.

With the shower being so effective at helping me cope, I wanted to try the bath. The midwife prepared the tub and I don't even remember the walk over to it. It was amazing to sink into the water, to feel the weight lifted off of my belly, and the warmth countering the pain. It seemed like I only had a few contractions here and then they started getting lower and stronger and a little overwhelming. Once again, the thought returned, "I can't do this much longer." The midwife walked into the room and I said to her, "I think I need to know how far along I am." She reassured me that my body was doing what it was supposed to and I was progressing well. She could tell that I wasn't comforted by this. "You'll start to feel pressure down in your rectum, you'll know".

I responded, "I do, I feel it all in my rectum".

Another surge came and I felt the urge to push, and I did a little bit, somewhat hesitantly, not knowing if it was time. "I feel something" I said frantically. One of the birth assistants came behind me to check as I was leaning over on the edge of the tub. "Oh, yes, that's your bag of water right there!" The midwife and the birth assistants realized how close I was and speedily prepared to help deliver my baby. Another surge, I pushed again and felt a shift. I can only assume it was his head moving down farther. The pressure was intense. "Can I push? I feel like I can push him out," I said somewhat frantically. "Wait for the contraction to build, but yes, he's right there Kennan, you can push now," said the midwife.

This is the moment I felt like I lost control. The pressure was more intense than anything I could have imagined and I was afraid, more than ever before, that I couldn't do this. I said it out loud for the first time, "I don't think I can do this". My husband and midwife responded quickly, "Yes you can, you already are, he's right there!" Elisha leaned closer, "Remember, Kennan, your body was made to do this." Another push and his head was born. Another push and quicker than I even realized what happened, my son was in my arms. A flood. An overwhelming flood of emotion. I'm not even sure I can list all of the emotions present. Joy, relief, love, amazement, thankfulness, awe. Knox was born at 5:54am, only 2 hours and 10 minutes after I'd arrived.

I had heard people say this and only half believed it, but it's true. The moment he was in my arms, all of the pain that had been all-consuming only moments before, meant nothing to me. It was comically trivial compared to the power and strength I felt. I labored for 9 hours total. I spent 2 hours at the birth center and pushed for only 10 minutes. I did it. My body did it. My birth was everything I dreamed of. I felt loved and empowered. Heard and respected. It was the most incredible experience of my entire life.

After my son was born, the tub was drained and they rinsed me off. The midwife and assistants helped move me to the bed. I delivered the placenta and got some stitches. I did have 2 first degree tears, probably because I was not super patient during pushing. Honestly, the stitches were worse than labor. This whole time we were doing skin to skin. After the stitches were placed, I breastfed my son for the first time. The birth assistants got my husband and I some snacks and we spent some time alone together. By 10:00am we were packing up to go back home. I couldn't believe they were actually letting us take him home. By 11:00am the three of us were in our home, starting our new lives together.

I am still amazed at the experience. I am in awe of my body and how perfectly it was designed to do this hard work. I am so thankful for my husband, I couldn't have done it without him. I am so in love with my son, Knox, who made me a Momma.

August 11, 2021

Kathleen and Madalyn

My birth is something I could relive over and over again. In the very early morning of August 10th, I was woken up by slight cramping a few times and I knew my body was starting to move towards labor. That morning I went about my normal daily routine – I took the dogs to the park, worked, worked out... In the late afternoon, things started to pick up and I was starting to feel the tightness intensify. I looked at my husband and said, "We will be having a baby in the next 24 hours." I knew things were progressing.

Around 4:00pm I called my midwives and told them that I thought I was in labor. They had me lay down to see if things slowed at all. While lying down, the contractions slowed a little but as soon as I stood back up, they picked back up. By 7:00 I could no longer talk through my contractions. So, we packed up and went to my midwife's home, which was thankfully only four blocks away. Riding in the car was quite the experience – one I would rather not have to do ever again.

We arrived around 8:00pm and were welcomed with open arms into a peaceful and beautiful space. My midwives, Marcy and McKenzie are the most wonderful humans. I worked through my contractions, moving from the couch to the floor and finally to the tub. Loren, my good friend and 'doula' arrived while I was trying to get comfortable. She supported me with conversation and hydration. Once I was in the tub, things progressed and so much pressure and discomfort were relieved. Between cracking jokes and chatting with my birth team, I was drawn into prayer, surrendering and working hard to give my baby girl the best birth possible. I kept telling my husband that I couldn't wait to go home and lay in bed with him and our baby girl.

At the point of transition, I was fighting back the dreaded throwing up. Marcy told me that throwing up was worth 10 contractions. I asked for the bucket and Loren came to the rescue. Once transition happened, I pushed for 2.5 hours. I wasn't tired, I just wanted to meet beautiful Madalyn. After almost 2 hours in the tub, I was told to move to the couch. Reluctantly, I got out and moved to the couch with a lot of help from my team. "I can't do this anymore!" I yelled. Then, three sets of pushes later, Madalyn Ann Granville arrived by flying out into Marcy's hands without a pause. The first person to talk to her was her daddy, and she got so quiet and just looked at him like she had known him forever.

I can honestly say I enjoyed the hard work it took to give birth. I can't remember the pain nor how intense it was, just the utter joy I felt the entire time knowing I was going to meet this perfect baby. The recovery and bonding have been a roller coaster and it's one I am ready to ride the rest of my life. I am beyond grateful for the opportunity to be her mom every day.

August 12, 2021

Jami and Baby O: A Birth in Texas

A supernatural labor and delivery is the only way to describe my birth with my son baby O. It was twelve hours from start to finish.

I am 40 weeks and 3 days…

My contractions started on Thursday morning at 6:00am. They were instantly about 5 minutes apart. The contractions continued to get closer and by 10:00am they were 2-3 minutes apart and I called my midwife. It was time to go to the birth center. I arrived around 11:00 and was 5.5 centimeters dilated and 100% effaced. I was ecstatic.

We got settled in our birth room and started to fill the tub. I labored on a ball for maybe an hour or so and had lunch – a Subway sandwich. Simple, but it tasted amazing at that moment. I had my headphones on and was playing a pumped up playlist to get me excited for birth. At this point time became obsolete. The next thing I remember was getting into the tub and I labored there until I started pushing. While in the tub I was rocking forward and backward to try and help lower the baby into my hips.

Once out of the tub, I sat on a birth stool because I felt pushy. My water broke and I moved to the bed. It was now about 5:00pm. I pushed on my back for about 30 minutes. Baby's heart rate skyrocketed to 200bpm. We prayed for my baby's heart rate to lower and that we would be able to deliver this baby safely. I got into an inversion to try and get the baby back out of the birth canal because he was the slightest bit stuck.

Another midwife came in about 20 minutes later. She reached in, adjusted baby's head, and then said, "With the next contraction, push as hard as you've ever pushed. We have to get your baby out."

With the next push his head came out. And the next his body came catapulting out of me.

Cue the tears of joy. At 6:21pm, baby O was born. He was healthy and happy. We are so grateful to our midwives in Katy, Texas for their education and skill. I wish any mom reading this is encouraged that they too can have a supernatural birth.

August 19, 2021

Rachel and Juniper Joy

5:22am: I had my first "real" contraction. I had another one 10 minutes later. I got up, went to the bathroom, and lost part of my mucus plug. I knew I was in the early stages of labor and I woke my husband up.

8:00am: I was still having contractions, so I called our midwife and she headed over. She stayed for about two hours to monitor them, but I didn't feel like my labor was progressing enough for her to stick around. She headed home and said to call when things got more intense.

10:30am: My mother-in-law took our older two kids with her for the afternoon. My husband and I went on a walk, ate lunch, hung out, and soaked up the last little bit of just us two.

1:00pm: My contractions were back to 6 minutes apart and felt more intense. Our midwife came back over. Juniper wasn't in the best position, so I tried to change into different positions during contractions. That really helped move her down to a better spot!

2:30pm: I felt a shift and decided it was time to get in the birth pool. The water gave me a lot of relief. I felt so peaceful and calm there. Every time I had a contraction, I closed my eyes, took deep breaths, and prayed. Every contraction was bringing me one step closer to meeting Junie.

3:05pm: I started to get super uncomfortable, so I changed positions. Instead of sitting, I leaned over the edge of the birth pool.

3:15pm: My water broke. It felt like something had popped! I knew it would be a matter of minutes before Juniper was here!

3:16pm: I delivered her head and really focused on not pushing so I wouldn't tear. I just breathed her down and out.

3:17pm: My midwife caught our girl and passed her to me. I literally shouted for joy! I couldn't believe what just happened!

After she was born, I got out of the tub and delivered the placenta. It was big and beautiful. We delayed cord clamping as long as it took to turn white, enjoyed some skin to skin, and she latched almost immediately. We introduced her to her siblings and settled into life as a family of five.

August 20, 2021

Anaïs and Daphnée: A Birth in Ontario, Canada

I had a hard time believing I was really in labor at 40 weeks and 3 days. I had been having very manageable prodromal labor for about a week prior. On August 20, my contractions began around 2:30pm while I was lounging in the pool with my family. Unlike the previous days, the contractions did not disappear once I got moving, although they did slow down a bit when I left to go get my toddler from daycare. By the time I returned home, contractions were about 5-10 minutes apart, 30 seconds long, but still very mild in intensity.

They felt different than they had with my first birth. They felt like an electrifying pressure starting in my core and expanding outward. They did not feel painful. I went about my evening as I usually would. Once my daughter was in bed, I felt my contractions pick up in intensity – they were now 2 minutes apart and 30-45 seconds long. However, because there was the odd contraction that was further apart, and they were not one minute long, I was telling myself I was not that far along.

We tried watching a movie, but I couldn't focus enough to enjoy it, so my husband suggested I go take a bath. Although with my first labour I had wanted no one to talk to me or touch me, I was happy to have my husband sit by me while I was in the tub. I got out after 30 minutes because we ran out of hot water. I headed downstairs and remember looking at the almost-full moon. It had a bright orange tinge to it. I looked at the time: it was shortly after 9:00pm and I told myself we would be having a baby likely the next morning. I was so excited!

My husband began setting up the birth pool and boiling water for it as we had no hot water. By this point, I finally realized that my contractions were coming regularly every 2 minutes. The intensity picked up again, although I would not describe them as painful as long as I swayed my hips and leaned over our counter during a contraction. With my first birth, I had had extremely long, double-peaking contractions, so this labour felt completely different. I had a hard time believing this was not still early labour. We decided to call the midwife around 9:25pm. She said she would be on her way immediately. My mother arrived shortly after as I wanted her there for the birth, too.

About 20 minutes later, I began feeling my body start to push during contractions. My husband said the midwife was still at least 25 minutes away. I gulped and tried to breathe through the contractions as best I could. I told myself if she wasn't here by 10:15pm, I would simply get in the pool. 10:15 arrived, and as I stepped into the pool, my midwife arrived, along with my sister who was there to take pictures. I asked if she wanted to check me, but she told me she trusted me and I could get in the pool if I wanted to.

Getting into the birth pool felt magical and instantly relaxed me. The first contraction I had in the birth pool resulted in my waters releasing. We heard a pop, and I looked back to see the fluid mixing with the pool water. Two minutes later, I started pushing. Two minutes later, another contraction began and I reached down and felt my baby's head come out. The rest of my baby came out with the following contraction, after only four minutes of pushing, at 10:29pm (and not the following morning as I had thought it would).

My husband couldn't wait to find out what we were having… and exclaimed that we had had another girl! We snuggled in the birth pool as I wrapped my mind around the shock of what had felt like a really quick birth. Her cord was extremely short, so we got out not too long after. I delivered the placenta at 10:47pm. The midwife explained that she had had a nuchal hand, which unfortunately resulted in a second degree tear. I didn't care – this birth had honestly felt pain free. Even though I had labored for 8 hours, it had taken me so long to believe it was really labor that I was still in shock that our baby was here! After getting stitched up, we went upstairs to snuggle for the night.

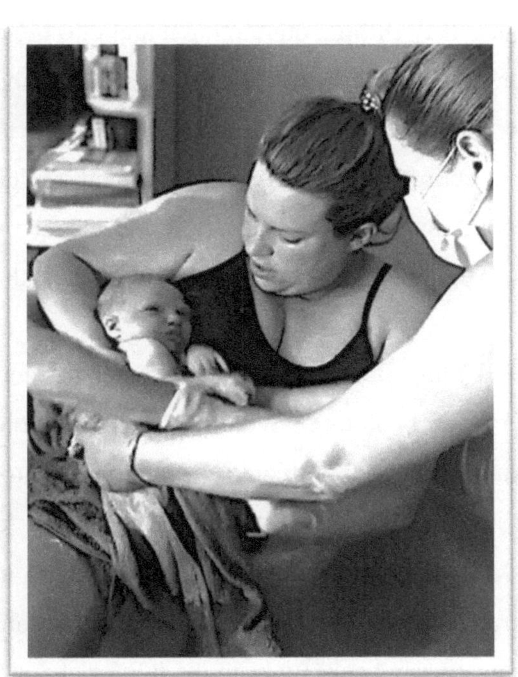

Megan and William

On August 20th, I had my 39-week prenatal appointment with my midwife at the birthing center. We talked about getting closer to my estimated due date and went home for it to storm the whole night. I had been having pretty strong Braxton hicks since the beginning of my pregnancy, so I figured that was what I was feeling that night. The contractions lasted all throughout the night and into the morning until around 6:00am. I got up because I felt like I needed to shower, and my water broke when I stood. I called the midwife and she told me to rest and count contractions, but I had back labor and couldn't really tell when they ended and started. I showered and cleaned up the house before my husband made me get in the car to head to the birth center in Nashville.

I stopped for breakfast first, and that's when my contractions got to the point I couldn't talk through them anymore. I got to the birthing center and was 4 centimeters dilated. I got straight into the tub. My midwife and her assistant were amazing! They were very hands off and showed my husband different ways to help with my back pain during a contraction. I spoke a bit in between contractions, but mainly rested to get my energy back. I was in the tub for about 4 hours when they asked if I wanted to switch positions. I had a few contractions on the toilet and tried a few on all fours, but it killed my back. I got on the birthing seat and that's when I was crowning, so I pushed for 20 minutes and as soon as he came out, he was placed on my chest. We waited for the cord to stop pulsing before my husband cut it. It was amazing! I was told I would be begging for drugs, but I wasn't! I could definitely tell when I was in transition, but I stuck to my birth plan, and it was amazing.

August 29, 2021

Sarah and Mira

My second baby girl was due to arrive on August 29th. Prodromal labour began 6 days prior, and each day I would get so excited and emotional thinking it may be the day I'd meet her, but also the last day with just my first baby. I had greatly considered having a home birth this time and figured I'd prepare for it, but make a final decision when the time came. The morning of August 28th, I woke up feeling extra crampy. I did the Miles circuit and went for a walk early in the morning. I noticed contractions became consistent and were 8-10 minutes apart. My instincts told me that active labour would be here soon, but I decided to distract myself as I didn't want to get my hopes and emotions up again just to have them crash back down.

I kept busy— I cut the grass, pulled weeds, did laundry, cleaned the house. We went to my parents' house for our usual Saturday night dinner. I enjoyed the company of my family while I took deep breaths through each contraction. They came consistently 7 minutes apart and lasted 40 seconds. Dinner came to an end, and I had to decide whether or not to leave my first baby with my parents or not. I followed my gut and said goodbye, but this was not without tears while driving away - it was our first time leaving her in her 2.5 years! As we were leaving, my dad said, "Something is telling me it'll be 2. 2:00am or 2:00pm, something to do with 2." I remember saying, "Well, it won't be 2:00am!" After all, my first labour was 48 hours… there was no way this baby would be here in 6 hours!

My husband and I got home and I had a shower, put my jammies on, and continued to do some things around the house. Around 10:00pm, contractions grew stronger in intensity but were still 7 minutes apart. Each time a contraction came, I began to lunge back and forth while holding onto something and breathing deeply. "Relaxed face, relaxed hands," I would remind myself. My husband put on Home Alone (Christmas movies are one of my greatest comfort measures) and I sat on my yoga ball to see if things would pick up or slow down. I told him to head to bed and get some rest. It was 11:00pm. He headed upstairs and within minutes, my contractions suddenly jumped from 7 minutes apart to 3 minutes apart. My husband was not getting the rest he had hoped for! I tried to wait an hour to call my midwives, but after 30 minutes the contractions were so intense, I knew it was go time. I called my midwife and just by talking to me she knew it was time. I decided to go to the hospital for the birth.

The whole car ride there, contractions were coming closer and closer together. We arrived and I could hardly walk. My husband kept reminding me, "Relaxed face, relaxed hands," with his soothing voice, while putting pressure on my back. He was the best doula I could ask for. We somehow got away without signing in or being screened for Covid; the hospital staff saw the state I was in, gave me a wheelchair, and sent us on our way. My husband literally RAN me to the L&D ward. I saw my midwife as we arrived and felt such relief to know I was in her care. She asked for my consent to be checked, which I agreed to. But not until after I threw up multiple times. Turns out, my midwife wasn't able to check me... baby was crowning! "Do you feel a bit pushy?" She asked. I think I responded by puking some more.

Things were happening so fast that they didn't have a room set up for me. Walking down the hallway, I was unsure if I'd even make it to the room. But I did! They asked if I wanted to get up on the bed. "No thanks... I can't move... I need to stand... I need to push..."

I gave one push while standing up. My waters broke and her head and hands came out. "Take a breath and try to wait before pushing again," my midwife said. I couldn't wait… baby pushed herself totally out on the second contraction. She was here! My midwife handed her to me. Pure bliss. I fell in love all over again. She was born on August 29 at 1:58am; just two minutes shy of 2:00. My dad was right!

Unlike my first birth, I felt some pain this time, even with those wonderful postpartum hormones rushing in. Turns out I had a pretty significant tear on my clitoris artery (due to baby girl coming out so fast with both hands up), which required some special attention. I'm sure I could've had a beautiful home birth, but part of me knows that this birth happened exactly the way it was supposed to.

August 30, 2021

Cynthia and Gaia

After 16 years, I forgot what a contraction felt like. I looked over to my husband as if he had an idea. It was Friday night and I was starting to feel something in my body that I couldn't describe yet. It was as if I had butterflies fluttering through my belly to my pelvis with a slight jolt every few hours. What was this? Was our prince or princess on their way earth side?

I was past 40 weeks and with non-traditional medical care, our hearts were at ease that our little one would come when ready. We opted out of ultrasounds during our entire pregnancy for personal and health reasons, so gender was a surprise. We were beyond excited, yet also quite exhausted since I had been very ill with flu like symptoms for the past couple weeks. In that moment, it was as if my body knew to focus on the baby and not on the illness.

Saturday came and our birth coach arrived to assist in our home birth. We tracked the contractions using an app. I ate delicious food made by my grandmother and had amazing snacks curated by my birth coach and hubby, including a scrumptious smoothie. It was heaven on earth. We had walks in the backyard in gorgeous sunny warm weather. We even had some time for a sweet intimate exchange, one last beautiful round of love before the baby arrived.

Sunday came along with contractions still going strong. I had very little sleep since Friday and was somewhat nauseous, but we kept the free flowing movement. Walked. Bounced. Danced. Talked. Ate. Took long and slow deep breaths.

It was time to prepare the birth pool and fill it with warm water to help ease the waves of labor. It was so helpful and such an amazing feeling being one with the water. It was simply beautiful. Waves came closer and closer. My husband grabbed my hand while I endured the waves of labor. My birth coach helped ease the pressure on my back. Warm towels. Gentle touch. Soothing sounds. Dim, calm and loving environment.

Monday morning came, and the birth coach stated it may be time to visit the hospital due to an irregular heartbeat of the baby and challenges with my cervix opening. At 4:00am, with no hospital bag pre-packed, we drove one physically painful drive to the only hospital in our area. I had to be in triage alone due to the pandemic restrictions. What seemed like forever, but was really an hour and a half later, my husband arrived for support. It felt cold and lonely to be in such a bright medical space coming from such a loving place - my home. We were prepared for whatever came our way as our birth coach talked us through every scenario she could think of.

It was a rather difficult experience to advocate for myself in a medical space where natural and unmedicated births were rarely seen. I clearly voiced my terms, my views, and my plan for what my birth would look like in this setting. Thankfully, our birth plan was respected. With waves of labor still coming, my husband's hand went numb from applying constant pressure on my lower back. During transition time and I felt every wave of discomfort and pain. I breathed heavily and allowed the sounds of labor to be heard by humming, moaning and practically screaming with the door wide open.

The nurse came in and placed the peanut ball between my legs. Within a few seconds of the next wave, my water broke, gushing forcefully onto the floor. It was as if a bucket of water was dumped. It was exciting yet terrifying. I tried to remember every hypnobirthing exercise and breathing technique, but in that moment, I was ready to push. The nurses expressed that I needed to wait to push, as if I could stop my body from what it was naturally preparing to do. I asked for support to help me squat, and I started pushing with no medical staff in sight.

Staff slowly came in and started setting up as I continued to grab my husband's hand for dear life. An amazing nurse helped get me into rhythm with my breathing to help with such an amazing and powerful birth. It was a few minutes later and all I remember was hearing, "It's a girl!" Looking at my husband as he was tearing up, I let the waterworks flow with such love and joy.

September

September 3, 2021

Tawny and Elias

At 40 weeks and 2 days, I woke at 12:15am and felt mild, annoying surges, just like I'd been experiencing for weeks. They were a little more uncomfortable than normal, but I chalked it up to dehydration. I decided to drink a glass of water and take a warm bath to try and relax. While in the bath, the surges continued and came regularly. At around 1:00am, I woke my boyfriend so that he could assemble and fill our birthing pool. This is when things got hectic.

Unfortunately, we did not do a practice-run of preparing the pool. It took some time to get it inflated and our hose adapter did not fit on our faucet correctly. Around 2:00am I called Kathy, my midwife, and she was confident that I was in active labor. She said she was on her way. I asked my aunt to come and help with the pool. She lives close and arrived almost immediately. My contractions were getting more intense and I decided to go to the bathtub for comfort.

Once in the bathtub, my surges were coming quickly, one after another. They were very intense. When my midwives arrived, one of them was able to use the water hook-up from our washing machine to begin filling the pool. I consented to a cervical check and was 7 centimeters dilated. They continued to fill the pool, using what little hot water we had left. They also started warming pots of water on the stove. I continued laboring through transition in the bathtub, holding onto my boyfriend through each surge and focusing on my breathing.

At one point my team assisted me out of the bathtub and into the pool in between surges. Once in the pool, surges were right on top of each other. I was shivering non-stop and was only comforted by the constant pouring of water on my lower back. I was laboring on my knees while leaning forward over the side of the pool, draped over my boyfriend's shoulders. Not long after getting into the pool, I began to feel my body pushing. I focused on relaxing my body to allow this reflex to take over. I added a little extra pushing to what my body was naturally doing on its own. I felt what I thought was the "ring of fire," but I didn't hear anyone say anything about the baby being here. In that moment I was scared to push and feel that pain again, until my midwife said, "Just one more push to get the shoulders out." Relief washed over me, knowing the worst of it was over and that my baby was here.

My son was born into the water at 4:43am and was immediately brought to my chest. He was perfect, calm, and not crying. His big brother woke up at some point during the commotion and was able to greet his new baby brother minutes after his birth. We spent our entire day snuggling our perfect 8 pound, 8 ounce addition. I had no idea that I was capable of such strength. Having my son at home was one of the best decisions I have ever made and left me with a lasting appreciation and passion for birth.

Jamie and Zoey

On August 24th I had an appointment with my midwife and mentioned I had been feeling a little itchy. I knew itchiness was a possible symptom of cholestasis because I had been tested for it during my first pregnancy. I had different symptoms then, and my test was thankfully negative My midwife suggested we establish a baseline with some bloodwork and go from there. She noted that results often took 10-14 days to come back, so the sooner we tested, the better.

At 5:40pm, on September 3rd, I received an email from the lab with my results. I did, in fact, have cholestasis this time. It hadn't really been on my mind since the appointment because the itchiness had let up. I immediately began researching what it meant for me and my baby. Most search results said mothers are routinely induced before 38 weeks due to the high risk of stillbirth.

My mind and heart began racing since I was 37.5 weeks along already. We had prayed and prepared to have another baby for years. Suddenly, in that moment, thinking I would need to deliver early was terrifying. I was overwhelmed with worry about our baby's safety as well as getting induced.

When my husband came home from work, I almost couldn't share the worrisome news. Soon enough, he noticed something was wrong. I broke down in tears and told him about the test results. He asked if my midwife knew, and wondered what she had said. I insisted she would get the same email and call soon. We waited all of 10 minutes to hear from her until I gave in and called her. I relayed my concerns, but she hadn't even received the results yet. We hung up so she could review them while my husband and I patiently waited. My phone rang shortly after, and my midwife explained the complications of cholestasis and went over my options:

Option A: Go to the hospital, get induced, and deliver that night.

Option B: Retest in a few days to see if the levels increased.

At that point, I plummeted into a deeper panic. I knew an induction would be likely, but I hadn't thought it would be that night. We made the decision that we needed to get the baby out. My midwife called the hospital to get us in for an induction, only to find out the hospital was completely full. We opted to go to another hospital and everything from then on moved quickly. I frantically gathered things to put in our hospital bag, while also packing my daughter's things for her first night away.

By the time we got to the hospital and settled into the delivery room, it was about 9:00pm. My midwife met us there with the sweetest nurse, Tammy. They hooked me up to a spider web of wires so I could be monitored because of the concerns that cholestasis presents for the baby. Shortly after, I started experiencing very frequent contractions on my own—which I hadn't been having at all before. It was as if my mental state had thrown my physical body into labor all on its own.

By 10:00pm I was started on a Pitocin IV drip to move things along. My contractions were becoming a little more intense, but nothing crazy, and I was told to get some sleep. I was too excited to sleep, so I laid there and waited anxiously, trying to pass the time. At about 1:30am my midwife came in and asked if I wanted her to break my water, since my contractions weren't getting any stronger. I said yes.

After my water was broken, my contractions went from 0-60 in an instant. I walked around and tried to move through them for a while. Then I decided to try the birthing tub. The contractions were so intense at this point. Knowing how long I was in labor with my first, my mind caved and I cried out that I couldn't do it anymore and I wanted an epidural! I sat there in the tub while I waited for the anesthesiologist. About three contractions later I said, "I need to poop!"

Again, I didn't think I was ready to have my baby this quick, since I had an extremely long labor with my first. Nurse Tammy had me get onto the bed so she could check me. I was dilated 8.5 centimeters and she called my midwife in. Just as she walked in, the anesthesiologist tried to come in, too. Before he even got through the threshold, both my midwife and Tammy shooed him away saying that I was ready to push the baby out. My heart sank. I was already in overwhelming pain, I was doubting my ability to continue on.

Once I got the hang of a good push, the pain from the contractions eased. It felt good to be able to push through the pain. I pushed for about 30 more minutes. Suddenly, a chunky baby girl shot out into this world and was laid on my chest at 4:25am. Our hearts doubled in size when we finally met our precious Zoey girl.

September 6, 2021

Katie and Layla Rose: A Birth in Massachusetts

It was a very long summer expecting the arrival of my last baby while chasing around a two and three-year-old. My daughter's due date was September 9th. Since this was not my first rodeo, I knew that her due date meant nothing. Babies come when they are ready. My other two children were both late. I was induced twelve days late with my daughter and went into labor on my own six days late with my son, who I delivered naturally.

I didn't hire a doula for this birth because I was unsure of what Covid restrictions might be in place at the time of delivery. It also wasn't that long ago that my son was born and I felt confident that my husband would be able to give me the support I needed. Heading into the Labor Day weekend I was having very mild contractions. We took the kids to the park, we went bowling and I kept pretty busy. I knew this baby would make her arrival before the long weekend was over.

Monday, September 6th arrived and we had our friends offer to take our two children so I could run errands and rest for the day. I took a nice solo trip to TJ Maxx and the grocery store. Once the kids were back home for nap time, my husband and I figured hey, let's have sex. So, we did that and then I took a nap. I woke up, the kids then woke up, and we started to figure out dinner. We decided to grill since it was a beautiful day in Massachusetts.

At 6:00pm I sat down to eat. Then pooof - I felt this drop as I sat down. Minutes later my contractions started. "Umm babe, you better call your Mom." My husband called his mom and asked her to head over to watch our kids. We knew it was time. At 6:45, my mother-in-law was still not at the house. My contractions were SO intense. I started bouncing on the yoga ball and pop – my water broke.

Around 7:00, my in-laws finally got to the house. We got in the car as fast as we could. We had a 25 minute drive into Boston where the hospital is located. Luckily, traffic was pretty light going into the city because of the holiday weekend. In my mind, I was thinking of all the hospitals we may need to go to on our way because this baby was coming out fast! The ride was not fun, but I was able to push the seat into my back and hips to help with the pain from the contractions. The seat provided some counter pressure to help me get through the drive.

At 7:35pm, we made it to the hospital. My husband left the car running and we walked into the hospital as I leaked an entire river of amniotic fluid on our way. It seemed like a 20 minute walk to get to

Labor and Delivery. We checked in and the nurse didn't even bother to triage me, she just got the room ready. I had my cervix checked when we got into our room and I was 9 centimeters dilated. I knew I could do this because I already had one natural birth and all the hard work was behind me at this point. Once the monitoring, Covid test, and blood work were done, it was basically time for me to push. After about six minutes of pushing, our daughter, with her full head of dark hair, entered the world. Layla Rose made it a Labor Day I will never ever forget.

September 6, 2021
Kristen and Emmie

On Thursday September 2nd I went in for a midwife appointment. I was 38 weeks and 4 days pregnant. We had some concerns with my baby's placenta after an ultrasound the week before said it was aged and a grade 4. We talked about that, and I asked to be checked since I had been having Braxton Hicks for weeks. My intuition was telling me we needed to deliver this girl soon.

When she checked me I was 3 centimeters dilated and 40% effaced. I was very happy. My blood pressure was a little high, but my urine was fine. My midwife also did a membrane sweep. We then discussed getting a follow up ultrasound on Monday and having daily monitoring to keep an eye on baby girl's heart rate. I left and started doing a lot of bouncing on a yoga ball and walking. I started losing some mucus plug and had some bloody show. That night I had some stronger contractions for about 3 hours, but as soon as I went to bed they stopped.

I saw my midwife again on Saturday the 4th and she checked me again. Now I was 4 centimeters dilated and 50% effaced. She did another membrane sweep. Baby had flipped to sunny side up, making it hard for her to get a good heart rate reading. I went home with her peanut ball and had instructions to do the Miles circuit with the ball and inversions to get her to flip back around. That night it was very quiet. I had real contractions and slept very well.

On Sunday the 5th, I went in to be monitored again. I was very anxious about getting her out. This time I was 5 centimeters and still 50% effaced. Baby girl had flipped back where she needed to be, but my blood pressure was still higher than normal. I had one last membrane sweep even though my midwife said there was not much more membrane to sweep at this point. I felt like we were close and that night I did some walking outside, bounced on my ball and took a dose of midwives' brew around 9:00pm.

By 9:30 I was having some light contractions. I started timing them at 10:30 and kept my midwife updated. These definitely felt different than previous Braxton Hicks, so I was hopeful that this maybe it. By 1:00am the contractions were more regular and very slowly getting stronger. My midwife wanted to come listen to baby, so she arrived at 2:00am and ended up just dozing on my couch. I stayed up and watched some TV and kept moving on my ball. I could not calm down enough to sleep.

At 5:30am things started to change. I was 6 centimeters and 70% effaced with bulging waters and my contractions increased in intensity. I woke Tyler up. I called my doula/photographer and had her come over. I have a big family and we all live in the same town. I called my mom, my four sisters, and my aunt to come over and hang out in the background.

My older three kids woke up around 7:00 and were fed and sent upstairs to watch some TV. I started to feel baby moving down and told the crew to hurry and set up the bed and birth pool. With each contraction the pressure in my butt was building. We moved into my room and literally as soon as the pool was filled, I had a contraction where I started to push. I jumped into the pool right around 8:00am. My body was pushing with every contraction. Every push I felt her moving down. I did not have much control of the pushing phase, but tried to slow it down when I felt her head starting to crown. As soon as her head was out, I felt her turn. Then I pushed with the next contraction to get her body out. She was struggling to get out, so I did the hardest push ever and she emerged into my arms. No tearing or stitches needed! She let out some grunts, but did not cry right away. You could tell by her breathing sounds that her lungs had a good bit of fluid to clear out.

When the placenta was birthed, I could tell it was abnormal. It was covered in calcification spots and had an extra lobe. My intuitions were right to get her out quickly. I'm not sure if the problems arose because I had Covid, but that is when they noticed a problem.

The midwife worked with my baby girl for about an hour to get all of the fluid out from her lungs and then she started screaming. She started nursing perfectly and is very loved by all.

September 8, 2021

Sandrine and Fiona

The morning of September 8th I woke up to a contraction. It was manageable, but noticeable. I had prodromal labor on and off for weeks, but this one felt different. As the day progressed, my contractions continued but were spaced far apart. After dinner, I tucked my first daughter into bed. I even read her a bedtime book while breathing through my contractions. Labor was ramping up and

I knew that this would be the last night as a family of three. As soon as she was in bed, full blown labor started. My contractions were immediately five minutes apart and they felt hard. My husband called our doula and she decided to pop over to see how I was doing.

My contractions were every three to five minutes, so we decided to call our birth team to come over as well. The midwife team and doula arrived around 9:00pm. Originally, I did not want any cervical checks during labor, but I needed to know where I was at. I got checked and was 4 centimeters dilated. The midwives let me continue laboring and said they would come and check on me in an hour. This labor was different from my first - I couldn't find labor land. I was too present in my surroundings. I was having a really hard time staying on top of my contractions and finding a rhythm. When the midwives checked me an hour later, I had barely dilated any more. We decided that everyone needed to leave so I could really focus on the contractions and labor.

Finally, I was able to go internally and really connect with my body. I created a little routine laboring on the toilet, in the shower, and leaning over my yoga ball. Whenever labor got too overwhelming, I would switch up my position. I loved the bath during my first labor but ended up absolutely hating it during this labor. Finally, around 6:00am, labor seemed to be changing and we decided to call everyone back to my house. I got checked again and now was 7 centimeters with contractions coming fast and furious. I reached the point where I felt like I couldn't do it anymore. It is an odd feeling - you feel so out of control, but your body is in control of everything happening. My water had not broken yet, so my midwife said we could see if it breaks on its own or she could break it for me to see if that would make things progress further. While I was trying to decide, my water broke on its own. It even made a loud pop noise.

At one point I was really struggling with my contractions. I was asking for help and trying to run away from my own body. My midwife suggested laboring on my side. I tried laying down and immediately hated it! I jumped out of bed as quickly as I could, and it felt like a bowling ball dropped in between my legs. I felt my baby drop into the birth canal. I told everyone that she was coming. My midwife suggested I try and touch her head to see where she was. It was one of the coolest feelings to have the power to check how close my baby was to being born. Nobody gave me permission to push, instead they told me to trust my body. I was upright, leaning over the edge of the bed, and my body took over.

After 30 minutes, I was tired of standing, so I got on my hands and knees. I felt her head coming out very slowly. Then everything became a little chaotic. Her head came out fast, but the rest did not follow. She was stuck. My midwife was so calm and handled everything so beautifully. She performed the Rubin maneuver where she reached up and rotated the baby's shoulder to get her unstuck. Within seconds of being freed, at 9:23am, my beautiful Fiona was born! Just like I expected, she was full of fire and let everyone know of her arrival. She was 8 pounds, 8 ounces of sweet squishy baby. She was almost two pounds bigger than her sister was at birth! Labor was a lot longer and harder than anticipated. The only surprise we did not have was that she was born on her actual due date. The beauty of a homebirth is that her big sister got to meet her immediately and we got to settle in as a family of four. I was so incredibly thankful for the knowledge and power my midwife team and doula held. They never showed fear and my birth was so beautiful!

Kelsey and Skylar

My labor with Skylar started on September 9th. It was the exact date that I predicted her to be born, and a week earlier than her estimated due date. When I saw that my work out for the day was snatches and doubleunders, I told my husband that this is a birthing day workout!

Shortly after returning home from working out, the Braxton hicks changed into very mild contractions. I rode them through the whole day and just stayed busy doing my normal house work and life with my 3 year old. We filled the day with friends, ice cream, pool time outside, and pulling weeds. My whole birth team, including my midwife, had a big sleepover because no one wanted to miss the birth in case it picked up quickly. I was able to sleep off and on through the night and woke up with no significant change in the morning.

As per tradition in our family, we drove to the beach for a walk. The 10th is my brother's birthday, so he joined us for the beach walk and lunch before I came home for a warm bath and a nap. When I woke up, I could tell that things were shifting. My daughter and I were watching tv when my water broke and contractions started. I called the midwife and my two friends who planned to attend the birth to notify them that it was time.

I set up my essential oil diffuser in the bathroom with my labor play list and got in the shower. It was a magical time as my baby was kicking and moving with me. I sang worship music and just reflected on how magnificent birth is. I was very comfortable there and just practiced moving my body to encourage baby down.

After a little while I decided to start laboring on my side in bed. This was my plan to try and stay relaxed and restful instead of trying to run from the discomfort. My friend took some family pictures for us, including my 3-year-old who was also present for the birth. I enjoyed chatting with everyone between contractions and practiced breathing and keeping my body open. When I was dilated to about 4 centimeters, it became more difficult to stay relaxed. At this point we cleared the room of everyone but my husband.

Transition felt hard and my mind went to a place of self-doubt and, "I don't ever want to do this again." I was able to reaffirm myself with the phrase, "I can and I will." My husband was the perfect birth support person, and he continued my music, massaged my back, and told me, "Just this one contraction, just breathe through this one." I transitioned from four centimeters to ten centimeters and was ready to push in about an hour. We brought everyone back into the room: my mom, my aunt, my two friends, and my daughter, as well as the midwife and her assistant. I pushed for 20 minutes on my side with my husband supporting my legs.

I had my hand on my baby's head from the minute she was crowning. From the corner of the room, I could hear my daughter say, "That's my baby!" Her words gave me all the strength that I needed to push my baby out. I grabbed her up and pulled her to me before the midwife could even catch her.

We named her Skylar Quinn and her sister cuddled right up with us and began showing her a baby book to catch her up on everything she had missed in life so far. It was truly a beautiful birth and it was so special to include so many of my favorite people. I love my midwife and her assistant, who rearranged her schedule to attend my birth as she did for my first. I would say to any mamma considering a natural birth that you are strong, wise, and you know how to birth your babies. Trust your instincts and they will take you far.

September 11, 2021

Samantha and Holden: A Birth in Upstate New York

We had tried for years to get pregnant. I did a bunch of testing and then reached the conclusion that I didn't ovulate on my own. We tried a few medicated cycles the summer before I got pregnant that were unsuccessful. I ended up getting pregnant naturally in December. None of the doctors could figure out what had worked, but we were so excited.

Because we had tried to get pregnant for so long, I had time to know what kind of birth I wanted. I knew going in that I wanted to avoid medication if I could handle it, but I wasn't going to be upset if I felt pain relief was needed.

At around 4:30am on September 10th, I was woken up by minor contractions. I had my 39-week appointment later that morning, so I figured I'd wait, since the contractions were not super frequent yet. Once I went in for my appointment, my doctor said I was definitely in labor, but it was super early, so I could go home for the time being. My house is only minutes away from the hospital. We went into the hospital later that night because my contractions were getting close together. I was sent back home and told to come back once I couldn't talk during a contraction. I went back to the hospital at 8:30am the next morning. I could still talk, but it was only curse words during contractions. I was admitted at that point.

While in the hospital, they had issues with the monitor reading my contractions. I am overweight and I think that was probably why. They said if they broke my water, they could put something internally to keep an eye on them. I believe it was an IUPC (Intrauterine Pressure Catheter). I was fine with that because I was getting impatient. At around 6:00pm they broke my water for me.

They kept periodically checking to see how dilated I was. I was around 8 centimeters when I told the nurse I felt like I needed to push. She told me to try and wait because she didn't want me to damage my cervix if it was not fully dilated. She had the doctor come in to check me and to get their opinion on what to do. The doctor told me it was time to push. Suddenly a bunch of people rushed into the room with equipment.

I pushed for about ten minutes and at 10:16pm he was born. I had minor tearing because my doctor was manually stretching me during every push. As soon as they put him on my chest, he grabbed my boyfriend's finger. Then he latched immediately. I absolutely loved the hospital where I gave birth. They never pushed a thing on us. If they suggested any interventions, they always gave us all of the information and let us make the decisions. I felt respected in my choices and am grateful for the happy hospital birth experience.

September 12, 2021

Kerstin April and Fiona: A Birth in Fiji

I learned I was pregnant only days before setting sail for the South Pacific. It wasn't planned that way, because we didn't expect to conceive the first time we tried on the solstice in December. I had enough time to buy prenatal vitamins, and not much time to process the news while busily preparing for an ocean voyage. My maternal grandma was in hospice, and I knew if I gave birth to a daughter, she would share my nana's name - Fiona.

I do not recommend sailing 2000 miles upwind during the first trimester. I truly love offshore sailing and usually never get sea sick, but this passage was not enjoyable at all. Seventeen days later, we arrived in a calm lagoon in French Polynesia and my energy and appetite instantly returned. My entire first trimester was spent sailing, surfing, freediving, and eating lots of fresh fish and coconuts. At 12 weeks, an American doctor sailed into the lagoon. She gave me an informal prenatal checkup, took my vitals, and checked my blood glucose and iron. At 20 weeks it was nearly time to sail to Fiji. I visited the village nurse for another checkup, just because it seemed like the right thing to do before sailing another 2000 miles. I got to hear my baby's heartbeat for the first time, and everything suddenly felt so real.

We arrived in Fiji at the beginning of my third trimester. I envisioned finding a local elder woman to serve as our birthkeeper, and was excited about the process. I began asking everyone I met if there was a wise woman in the village that would attend our home birth. To my surprise, the answer was unanimous: "Why would you want to do that? We give birth at the hospital now." I visited the midwife clinic at the hospital to ask if anyone there would attend a homebirth. The answer was the same. The midwives were all very pleasant women trained to Australian midwifery standards, but the resources and facilities in the hospital were severely lacking. There was no way I would be comfortable birthing there.

I began to realize that the Fijian culture has become very accustomed to following the direction of the western world. They considered the shift from home birth to hospital birth (no matter how poor the facility) as societal progress. I popped into the clinic another time to ask again, and got roped into an ultrasound that I didn't want. I figured if we found someone to attend the birth at home, it would ease their concerns to know I've done a few of the recommended things. The ultrasound machine was an old hand-me-down from Australia, and the technician said I was measuring 2 weeks behind and that my due date must be off. My husband was with me this time, and he was appalled at the state of the hospital facilities. We needed to find an underground midwife, or we would be free birthing.

I continued asking every woman I met if she had a friend or family member that would attend our birth, and I started using social media to post inquiries in every outlet I could think of - sailing groups, expat groups, community groups. I also continued to educate myself on physiological birth and made it my full-time job to ensure that my baby was positioned ideally for a smooth birth. I used a lot of "Spinning Babies" postures and exercises. I was preparing myself mentally, physically, and spiritually to potentially free birth, in case we couldn't find the right woman to join our birth team. In the meantime, we were still sailing and surfing. We also hoped that the border would open, and flights would resume, so that my mom could fly in to help us during labor and postpartum.

I met an American and South African expat couple at the marina bar who owned a vacation rental, and they offered us a discounted 1-month rental so we could birth in a home and have time off the boat during my immediate postpartum. The house was on a hillside, at the top of 100 steps, overlooking the bay where our boat was anchored. It was perfect. We were thrilled with the arrangement and felt that having a house to birth in would help make whoever was going to attend the birth more comfortable also.

Stories travel quickly around small tropical islands, and my situation became widely known. I got the name of a retired Fijian midwife, Ateca, and reached out to her to ask if she would meet with me to talk about my birth plan. We met at the same marina bar. She had delivered probably 75 percent of the adults on the island, and had studied midwifery in Australia, where she attended home births and water births. She understood my desire for a peaceful home birth and wanted to support me. She was also concerned that she could get in trouble with the government since she was no longer licensed. I asked her if she could attend the birth in a doula role because that was ideally what I wanted- a wise woman present to observe and offer guidance if I needed it.

In the final week of my pregnancy, Ateca managed to use her relationship with the hospital to convince the board of directors to allow one of the licensed midwives to attend my birth with her. This arrangement made Ateca more comfortable, and I agreed that all members of the birth team needed to feel comfortable for us to have the most relaxed energy and a positive experience. I was able to meet with Flori, the licensed midwife, to discuss my birth plan in detail, and explain that all she really needed to do was observe. I had to write a letter to the hospital directors stating that I was going against medical advice by giving birth at home and that I assumed all responsibility for any negative outcome.

On my due date, I spent a lot of the day in the pool, and I took two trips down and back up the 100 steps to our birth house. I went to bed at a normal hour with zero indications that my baby was ready to arrive. I was feeling well enough to believe that the baby could stay put for another two weeks. It rained heavily that night and I slept lightly- as I always did on a squally night at anchor, even though I was in a house. A sudden trickle of water from my vagina woke me fully. I managed to hold it back as I waddled to the toilet. Was it urine? Did my water just break? It definitely was not urine. Intermittent trickles kept coming, seemingly every time right after I changed my period panties. I checked the time- it was 3:30am, and I had a recent text from Flori (she was working a shift at the hospital from 7:00pm-7:00am). I told her I thought my waters were leaking, and I was going to go back to bed.

The frequent squirts of liquid kept me awake and then I suddenly had to empty my bowels. A few minutes later I needed to use the toilet again, and decided to head to the downstairs bathroom. I began feeling period-like cramps while sitting on the toilet. I knew I should try to sleep, but I ended up emptying my bowels two more times, and each time the cramping got stronger afterwards. I went up and down the stairs inside the house, eating a few dates in the kitchen upstairs, and sitting on the toilet downstairs. By the time the birds were waking and dawn was breaking, I knew that baby would be arriving that day. I used my doppler to listen to the baby's heartbeat, and it was steady at 150, just as it had been for weeks. I woke my husband up around 6:00am and told him it was baby day!

By 7:00am I was breathing through the surges. I used yoga and freediving breathing techniques while imagining my uterus receiving an abundance of oxygenated blood each time. I would inhale and then visualize my cervix relaxing and dilating each time I exhaled. I called Ateca to let her know that today was the day and that I felt like things were moving along efficiently. She said she would get herself ready and she would stop by the hospital on her way over to pick up Flori with her birth kit.

The midwives arrived around 10:00am. I was walking and talking, but pausing to breathe during surges. They observed me while we chatted, and they felt confident that I was in active labor. Everyone knew my birth plan in advance - leave me alone except to occasionally listen to heart tones with the doppler that I had purchased. The walls of the master bedroom didn't go all the way to the vaulted ceiling, so it was easy for the midwives to listen from the living room while I labored in the bedroom alone or with my husband. Surges were coming frequently and lasting close to a minute. Flori asked if she could check my cervix. I had stated in my birth plan that I did not want any cervical checks unless I asked for one, but at this point I was actually curious, so I consented.

Lying on my back was so uncomfortable, and the sensation of the surges in that position was so awful, that I immediately regretted the decision. The news that my cervix was 4-5 centimeters dilated almost disappointed me, until I remembered why I didn't want any cervical checks in the first place. They are not a true indication of how labor will continue to progress. Flori was sweet and well educated, but she was a medically trained midwife. She proceeded to inform me that I would likely be fully dilated by 3:30pm. I shook my head, "No," and told her, "No numbers, No time schedules." After that, I fully zoned out and only focused on using my breath to stay oxygenated and open up.

I didn't get back up after the cervical check. I just rolled onto my left side to rest and conserve my energy. I fully lost track of time and ventured deep into labor land. I hadn't eaten except for a few dates before sunrise, and I had no desire to eat anything. I could hear the midwives telling my husband that I needed to eat something. I said, "no" a few times, and eventually had one bite of papaya to appease everyone. I vomited with the next surge after eating just one bite.

The surges began emanating from my uterus through my pelvis and into my thighs. I was still lying on my left side, and I needed my husband to squeeze my right thigh as hard as he could during each surge. Experiencing this sensation in the bones of my thighs was actually the most difficult part of labor. In retrospect this was my transition phase, and my pelvis was opening.

At 3:30pm Flori wanted to check to see if I was fully dilated. I begrudgingly agreed, and asked her not to tell me the number. Again, I was extremely uncomfortable and borderline in pain while on my back during a surge. She left the room and my husband came in and told me I was completely dilated, and the midwives said I could push. I had zero urge to push. I wanted my body to tell me when it was time, not a number, and I definitely did not want to be coached to push. The midwives left me to labor for 3 more hours fully dilated- I had no idea of how much time had passed, though I did notice the daylight dimming.

The surges were still intense in my thighs, and I was waiting for my body to tell me it was time to push. I could hear the midwives saying they thought I was too tired. I realized they were probably thinking I would need to transfer, but there was no way I would let that happen. I tried a little push with the next surge and I could feel what felt like a water balloon coming out of my vagina. The amniotic sac was still intact and my baby's head was right there.

I knew I wanted to birth upright. I squatted on the floor at the end of the bed and held onto my husband's arms for balance and leverage. After a couple of pushes with the surges, the midwives told me I wasn't pushing correctly. I was still focusing my breath on relaxing and opening, and they told me I needed to hold my breath and push like I'm pooping. None of that advice felt right to me, but they were both far more experienced in birthing than me, so I tried it their way for the next surge. Each time I pushed the sac would bulge out and then suck back in after the surge. I asked to rupture the sac membrane, thinking it would help me to feel more "pushy."

We listened to heart tones before and after releasing the membrane's fluids and baby was doing great. I now felt a lot more serious about it being time to birth my baby. With the next few surges, as I felt the sensation coming on, I took a deep breath in and out and then a second deep breath in and held it while pushing. My body responded by pushing with me. I was able to put in 2-3 pushes during a surge, and after only a few surges, my baby's head was crowning.

The crowning surge faded before baby's head was fully born, and I pushed on my own to birth the rest of the head before the next surge. I was still squatting on the floor with my husband in front of me, and it was hard for the midwives to see what was going on. They asked me to get onto the bed, and my husband helped me get up and lay on the bed on my side. Flori moved the nuchal cord as I was laying down, and then told me I could push baby out the rest of the way. Baby's body birthed easily with the next surge and I was suddenly holding a tiny being on my chest.

It let out the tiniest cry and then was quiet and just looking around at us with big, beautiful eyes. I kept saying, "We did it!" to my baby, and then looked at my husband and said, "I could do that again." A few minutes passed before we checked to find out that I birthed a tiny baby girl. It was Fiona all along. We didn't have a scale, but the next day we used a baking scale and she was 5 pounds, 12 ounces, or 2.6kg. Born at 7:21 pm, at "home" in Fiji.

We let the cord go white and limp before cutting it. My husband had to drive Flori back to the hospital for her night shift that she was now late for. Ateca stayed with me and I birthed the placenta after about 40 minutes while sitting on a short stool in the bathtub with Fiona latched at my breast. By the time my husband got back from dropping Flori off at work, I was showered and in bed nursing our little girl. He brought some food to bed and crawled in with us. My world felt so complete, and I felt at that moment that if more babies could be born like this, the world could be a better place.

September 15, 2021

Kaysee and Nora

This was my second pregnancy and second home birth. I've always had the easiest pregnancies, but two weeks before my due date I was having prodromal labor and I was pretty over it by the end. The day before my due date, my midwife performed a membrane sweep. I had never had one before and my partner and I went home thinking labor would happen quickly, even though our midwife had told us it could take up to 24 hours.

The day went by and of course…no baby.

The next morning we still had absolutely no signs of true labor. I was in a full blown pity party. My dad had even called to check in and see if there was a baby and I was so annoyed when I had to say no. My partner came home on his lunch break around 11:30 and made my oldest and I some lunch.

About five minutes after finishing lunch, I had to go to the bathroom and I lost my mucus plug. It was exciting! But I was still not convinced the baby was coming. I texted my midwife and told her the news and she said to keep her updated. I laid back down in bed when five minutes later I had to go to the bathroom again. This time it was coming out the back end and it was coming out with vengeance. I laid back down again and then repeated the process three more times. I decided I couldn't leave the toilet. It was becoming more painful, but I was still not convinced I was in labor. At this point my partner decided he was going to start prepping things and told his work he was not coming back for the afternoon. The pain increased and I finally decided to call my midwife because I honestly couldn't stop pooping and needed help. She told me immediately that she was on her way!

It turned into total chaos. My partner was trying to set up the house how I wanted for my birth wishes. He was simultaneously running into the bathroom to comfort me. I didn't know if I was having contractions because I couldn't stop pooping. Instinctively something told me to go back to the bathroom. I dropped to all fours and immediately knew I was in labor. I could feel each contraction. They were coming every minute and a half and my midwife hadn't made it yet. My partner started trying to set up our birth tub when the midwife assistant walked in.

I had never been more relieved. She walked in with such calmness. "Hi Kaysee, how are you doing? Is it ok if I check you to see what's going on?" I always loved that they ask permission for everything. She immediately started going to work QUICK. She told my partner to stop trying to set up the tub because we didn't have time. Baby was coming NOW. She was also our birth photographer and she snapped photos, set up supplies, kept me calm, snapped more photos, and prepared to catch the baby.

Then I felt the head! She reassured me, "Yes Kaysee, if you give me one good push she will be out." I gave one strong push and just like that the head was out. After one more push, she was completely out! My midwife walked in about five minutes later. This entire birth took 40 minutes from start to finish! Man oh man, do I love home births!

Lora and Cedric

The clock ticked past two in the morning when I felt the most powerful surge of my pregnancy. I knew it was time. I had prepared all of the birth supplies weeks before in the spare bedroom, all I had to do was breathe and wait. Flickering candles lit the room as I filled the diffuser with essential oils and started rocking back and forth on the yoga ball. The only sound I could hear was my breathing and moaning, along with the hypnobirthing track I had been listening to since the second trimester.

In between contractions I would remind myself: Water. Rest. Breathe. Repeat. When I felt the surges coming very quickly, one after another, I made my way to the bathroom and squatted over the toilet. To mine and my husband's surprise, we could see and feel something going in and out with every surge, and we knew we had to be close. Another surge later and I leaped off the toilet. My water bag had burst all over the bathroom, myself, and my husband. I laughed at the mess, but was quickly brought back into labor with another surge.

This time I fell to my knees in the hallway, and I let out the biggest roar I've ever heard. Then everything fell silent, and something whispered, "It's time to let go of control. It's time to let go." I had prepared for this birth since before I was pregnant. I made sure to read every piece of information I could find on having a freebirth. But now something felt off, something shifted. I had to let go of having everything the way I had perfectly planned. I looked up at my husband and said, "Never mind about the homebirth, I need to get to the hospital. Something doesn't feel right."

We gathered what we needed to check into a hospital, and off we went. After twenty minutes in the car, I had lost so much fluid. I soaked my maxi pad, the clothes I had on, and the passenger seat. After endless questions about the entire duration of pregnancy to now, the nurse came in and asked if I wanted an epidural for pain. I looked at the entire staff in front of me, which looked like ten people. I said, "I don't need you to save me, I need you to save my baby! Something doesn't feel right!"

I was sitting on the edge of the bed when the on-call OB came in and said to lie on my back so she could do an exam. I rolled my eyes at the thought of something going in when I was trying to get something out. I climbed onto the bed and said, "I am not comfortable in that position, but I will do hands and knees." Another surge came and I instinctively went down to my chest and knees, then immediately back up to hands and knees. I yelled out, "Ring of fire! Ring of fire!" After another minute or so, this beautiful baby boy emerged. He was so silent, not a sound.

Everyone frantically tried to get different supplies, and so many people surrounded my baby. The NICU nurse handed him to me and quickly said, "He has meconium in his lung and it's collapsing. We have to get him upstairs, so you can only hold him for a second." Before I knew it, I was postpartum, sitting in a hospital bed, without my baby.

After five days, a million visits to the hospital, endless pumping, and less than eight hours of sleep, I would finally take my miracle baby home. The amazing thing about the entire experience is the transformation I felt within me. I had empowered and educated myself for a homebirth, then a freebirth, and finally advocated for myself and my baby with a hospital birth. The oxytocin must have kicked in big time, because I never felt so elated like I did at that moment in time.

Invincible, evolved, and so in tune - because I surrendered and believed in myself to do all the right things for me and my baby.

September 17, 2021

Christina and Logan

I made the decision to have an unmedicated home birth before Logan was conceived. We drove 1 hour to see my midwife for my monthly checkups. On the morning of September 17th, at 3:45am, I started getting somewhat regular pressure waves (contractions). I called my midwife, pretty sure they were not Braxton Hicks, and informed her. She told me to take off from work for the day. Much to everyone's surprise, Logan arrived 12 hours later.

My midwife told me to take it easy and start timing my pressure waves. My husband was home with me, and he got the birthing pool ready while I sat on the couch and read a book. My aunt, who was also my doula, arrived not long after my initial waves started and helped me through each one. I used my birthing ball to breathe through each sensation. At 1:45pm I decided to sit in the birthing pool for 20 minutes. I think this time in the water is what helped me relax enough to progress into transition. From then on everything went very fast. I went to the bathroom and lost my mucus plug and then proceeded to vomit. After this I went to lay on my bed. I breathed through the waves, which had become increasingly powerful. I was ready. I knew that I was ready to push. My midwife pulled in the driveway just as my water broke. In hindsight, I probably should have called her sooner, but she made it in time!

The midwife rushed into the room and checked my dilation. She told me to start pushing. What a relief that was! Logan arrived about an hour later. I can honestly say the worst part was the ring of fire, but my hypnobirthing and breathing helped me get through the discomfort of crowning. After his head and shoulders came through, it was easy.

The experience was amazing! I cannot wait to give birth to my future children in the comfort of my own home.

September 21, 2021

Alexandra and Sunday

At 39 weeks and 3 days, I began to have contractions that were very manageable throughout the day. At 5:00pm they started to get more intense. My husband was gone for an hour while he went to drop off a meal to a family that just had a baby a week earlier. When he got home, we called our midwife to let her know that active labor had begun. I was vocal through contractions, but I did not think my baby would be born anytime soon, as my previous labors had lasted about 8 hours.

About an hour after my husband got home from delivering the meal, we tried to fill the birth pool. We had to call a neighbor to help because I couldn't help through my contractions. My midwife arrived at 7:00pm. I felt like I had to poop so I sat on the toilet and yelled, "ITS NOT POOP!" I was guided back into the birth pool to birth my beautiful baby girl at 7:30. It was the most redemptive birth! It was so quick and beautiful!

September 25, 2021

Natalie and Julia: A Birth in California

From September 2019 to October 2020, I experienced three miscarriages. This was confusing after having three perfectly healthy, full-term pregnancies and beautiful home-births. My second miscarriage was an ectopic pregnancy that took two trips to the emergency room, one trip to urgent care, and multiple doctor visits before I was correctly diagnosed and given the emergency surgery I needed. At almost 38 years old with only one tube, I thought my chances of getting pregnant were pretty slim. After two years of trying and three losses, my husband and I were done. We decided to focus on gratitude and contentment with our three beautiful children.

Two months after my last miscarriage, I was waiting for period. Since we hadn't been trying anymore, and I only had one tube, pregnancy was completely off my radar. But sure enough, as soon as I peed on the stick, it was positive. I was overwhelmed with emotion. I was so excited and also so worried I would miscarry again. I had a sense of peace with this pregnancy, and I decided to not seek any care or tell my OB that I was expecting again. I had decided that one of three things would happen: I would have another early miscarriage, I would have pain and seek care for another ectopic, or I would grow a healthy baby. So I didn't seek any care until I was at the end of my first trimester.

As my pregnancy continued, I felt good. I loved being pregnant! My husband and kids were overjoyed. We decided to find out the gender (the other three had been surprises) and once we knew it was a girl, I couldn't believe how blessed I was to have two boys and two girls! My first was born 12 days late, my second was born 10 days late and my third came on his due date. I had a gut feeling baby number four would be at least a week late, but I was trying to be prepared for anything.

I was due Labor Day weekend, but the holiday weekend passed and there was no sign of labor. Another week went by and I was 41 weeks. I was determined to trust my body and was not interested in any natural forms of induction, so we just continued along. Another week went by and I was 42 weeks. I had never gone this long in pregnancy and the mind games were starting. The pressure felt high. My husband was trying to rearrange his work schedule; my midwife, Katie, had a huge family vacation planned to Hawaii coming up; my best friend, Sheridan (who was planning to be at my birth), had a trip to San Diego planned for her son's birthday. We were also entering an area of potential legal issues since there are somewhat strict rules around home birth in California! I needed to have this baby soon!

But as you know, stress and pressure don't make you go into labor, so I started looking at my options. As my midwife's vacation approached, we started talking about our backup plan. I decided to get a biophysical profile done to check on the baby. She and I had been doing great at my visits, but having an ultrasound felt valuable for the midwives taking over my care. She was perfect on the ultrasound, measuring about 8 pounds and looking like a 38 week baby. She had good fluid and passed all the tests within the first 10 minutes. She was happy and healthy. We looked at my dates again, and if we calculated from my positive pregnancy test, I was 42 weeks. If we went off my cycle, I would be closer to 43 weeks! But our baby girl was small and looked like a 38 week baby. We were confused, but also trusted the process and were reassured by her constant movement.

I decided to do some acupuncture and increase my chiropractic visits. I requested a vaginal exam during one of my midwife visits. I was not dilated much, but she was able to strip my membranes. Nothing worked.

Eventually it was Friday. On Saturday I would be 43 weeks, Katie would be on a plane to Hawaii, and my best friend would be in San Diego. It felt like I might be pregnant forever. Ironically, I was still feeling great and truly loved being pregnant. I wasn't sure I wanted it to be over.

I had my final prenatal visit with Katie on Friday afternoon. She was available until 4:00am, and then would be at the airport. My best friend got in her car and started driving to San Diego. Evening came and my parents came over to watch a movie with the kids while Craig and I went walking downtown. As we walked around, I started having some light contractions. I wasn't getting excited yet, but I was feeling encouraged. The light contractions continued, and I let my best friend know that something might be happening, but not to come back home yet.

I headed to bed around 11:00pm. At midnight I woke to a contraction that was firm enough to wake me, but not super strong. At 1:00am a contraction woke me up. I breathed through it and went back to sleep. At 2:00am a contraction woke me again, a little stronger, but nothing too intense. I went back to sleep. At 3:00am there was another contraction. This time I decided to let my midwife, the new midwife team, and my best friend know that I had been having consistent contractions, once an hour. I told them all that I assumed they would disappear in the morning.

I went back to bed and awoke with a contraction - it was 3:15am. Then I had another at 3:30, 3:45, and 4:00. I texted everyone again letting them know that they were now 15 minutes apart, but that I was sure they would not continue once the sun was up.

That 4:00am text was enough for my best friend to get in her car and start the 2 hour drive back home. She arrived around 6:30 and found me sitting in my living room breathing through contractions.

We decided to take a walk and get some breakfast and smoothies. My husband loaded the three kids in the car and headed out to my son's first cross country meet. He told us to text if we needed him. Our walk was on the slower side. I needed to pause and breathe when a contraction would come, but I continued to insist that they were not strong and would probably disappear soon.

We got back from our walk at 8:45am. I put my feet up and decided I needed a rest. I would doze off for a few minutes and then wake to a contraction. Sheridan had been timing my contractions and knew they were getting closer and consistent, but in my head, we were still in early labor.

By 10:30 I decided I wanted to take a hot shower. I stood and let the hot water run over my belly. With every contraction I breathed and focused on letting go, giving in, and relaxing as much as possible. I felt like I was in the shower forever. When I finally got out, Sheridan asked if I had had any contractions while in the shower. "Yes," I told her, "probably 4 or 5. Maybe 6." Her eyes got big and she told me I had only been in the shower for 20 minutes and we should probably let the midwife know.

Our backup midwife lived just 8 houses away, so we called her and she walked down the street to check on me. By this point my husband had filled the birth tub in the kitchen, the same place I delivered my other three kids. He also had snacks and water for me and had dropped our boys off with my dad at his home down the street.

My midwife and birth photographer arrived at 12:15pm and found me standing in my underwear leaning over my bed. I was swaying, breathing and telling myself, "It's not pain, it's pleasure." I was forcing myself to smile through the contractions, working to trick my brain into thinking this was not painful. I would rub my temple and jaw and recite, "Let it go." The contractions were strong, but I was managing them well. The midwife waited for my contraction to end before making any noise. She gently asked how I was doing and took my vitals. After the next contraction she listened to the baby with the Doppler. The baby sounded great!

I continued to labor leaning over my bed, smiling and rocking until I got in the birth tub at 12:34pm. My daughter, Kylie, almost 10 years old, was right by my side the whole time. She had watched her brother being born 3.5 years earlier and this time she wanted to catch the baby. We had talked a lot about labor and what to expect and we watched birth videos and discussed our plan for this birth. She was planning to be in the tub with me to catch her sister, while daddy and the boys watched from around the tub. Once I was in the water, Kylie was my little doula, she got me water, held my hand, rubbed my arm. She quietly observed me as I worked hard through each contraction. Craig sat with me as well, rubbing my shoulders, encouraging me and holding my hand.

A little after 1:00pm, the rest of the midwife team arrived. They quietly set up for the birth. About every 15 minutes one of them would come and quietly listen to the baby's heart rate after my contraction ended. She always sounded great.

At 1:15pm Karen arrived. I cried. Here is what you need to know about Karen… I met Karen when I was 20 weeks pregnant with my first baby. She was a local midwife we had decided to interview since we thought we might want a home birth. At the time I was a labor and delivery nurse at a high-risk hospital. I saw a lot of scary things, but also had a deep trust in my body and what it was capable of. Karen, as the experienced midwife that she was, helped me work through and overcome all the questions and fears I had around birth. Craig and I loved the care we received from her and we trusted her.

We had an amazing home birth with Kylie and hired Karen again for my next two pregnancies. During my year of miscarriages, Karen retired. She was still involved in the birth world, teaching student midwives, but not taking on any clients. When I got pregnant with this sweet rainbow baby, I struggled knowing that I would not receive care from Karen. The amazing midwife I hired, Katie, had trained under Karen and could consult with her if we needed anything, but it was just not the same as having Karen there to walk me through my pregnancy.

As part of the "back-up" plan, Katie had reached out to Karen to ask her if she would be willing to attend my birth if I went into labor while she was in Hawaii. Karen had agreed. At 1:15pm Karen walked in, and I cried. I had not seen her in over 3 years, but in that moment, it was as if no time had passed. It was so comforting to see her smile and hear her voice. It felt like everything was as it should be for me to have my baby.

I continued to contract every 4-5 minutes. They were strong and long but I was not feeling any pressure or urge to push yet. I asked Craig when his family would arrive. My mother-in-law is a very special person to me, and she had been at two of my previous births, along with my mother. My mom had arrived earlier in the day, but I was hopeful my mother-in-law would make it in time. They got stuck in traffic, but finally walked in the door at 2:43pm. I checked myself and could feel the baby's head, but it was not very low at all. As my mother-in-law came in to greet me, Craig and Sheridan stepped away. Sheridan went to the living room to greet my sister-in-laws and chat with the midwives that were all sitting and visiting.

"She waited for me!" my mother-in-law said, and she kissed my cheek. I started to have another contraction. I was leaning over the side of the tub, letting my belly hang in the water as I rested on my knees. As my contraction peaked, I felt the baby shoot down. I started grunting – LOUD. Then my water broke and I told Kylie to get in the water. Before the midwives could get in the room, before Sheridan could get her camera on, before we could get the boys from my parents' house, she was here! Julia was here! She shot out of me at 2:45pm. Kylie jumped into the water as Craig leaned over the side of the tub to catch.

Julia came out with lots of meconium and the water was immediately an interesting shade of yellow/brown. The cord was around her neck at least three times. Craig and Kylie carefully spun her under the water, unwrapping her from her very long cord. Kylie slowly pulled her up out of the water as I swung my leg over and turned around to see them. Kylie handed me my tiny rainbow baby. Her eyes were open, her lips puckered, and she had meconium staining on the side of her head. She hadn't taken her first breath yet. She looked at me as if to say "Wow, what was that?!" She had a line across her forehead, it looked like she had been sitting with my cervix like a crown for a while. I talked to her, encouraging her to take a breath. Everyone was around the tub, watching her, waiting to hear the first cry.

There was a mix of excitement and anxiety as we watched her close her eyes and become more limp. The cord was still pulsing, so we knew she was getting some oxygen, but her lips were still purple and she had not taken a breath. I gently blew on her face and encouraged her. About two minutes after she had been forcefully expelled, she still had not taken a breath. I was rubbing her gently as she tried to transition. The resuscitation gear was available, but not needed yet. She started to get floppy and in a calm voice, Karen told me to, "Give her a little puff." I put my mouth over her nose and mouth and gave her a little puff. After three slow puffs, she was still not responding. One of the midwives helped me to tip her upside-down in a draining position. She coughed, and at 2 minutes and 39 seconds old, she cried. There was laughter and sighs of relief. She immediately started to pink up and started moving her arms and legs. I lowered her back into the warm water and continued to keep a close eye on her.

We planned to have the boys there to watch the birth, but it happened so fast they missed it. Over the next 10 minutes we continued to rub her back, move her in and out of a draining position, and I gave her a couple more puffs of air to help move the fluid that was still in her lungs.

Exactly ten minutes after she was born, the boys walked in and got to meet her. She was calm and just looking around the room. She would respond to her siblings' voices, it was so sweet. Kylie got out of the pool. By this point my placenta was starting to release and there was a lot of blood in the water. At 3:16, Cooper (our second oldest) cut the cord and we handed baby Julia to her big sister while I squatted and worked on delivering the placenta.

By 3:25 I was climbing into our bed, Julia was having her first feeding, and Cooper was reading her her first book. After being looked over by the midwives, we moved out to the living room where all the family gathered around as Julia got her newborn exam. Every step of her exam was talked through, the big kids got to participate, and Craig got to weigh her. She was 7 pounds, 4 ounces - my smallest by over a pound and my latest at 43 weeks! After the exam, we "took a tour" of the placenta and showed the kids every part of the baby's home in my belly. Over the next few hours, we all soaked in sweet newborn snuggles and reflected on the amazing day.

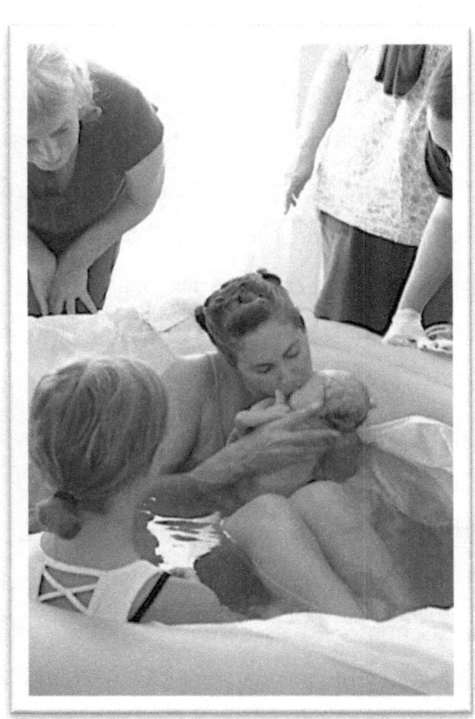

Abbey and Beckham

I had planned for a natural birth and practiced hypnobabies techniques to prepare. For two weeks I had prodromal labor with constant back pain and abdominal cramping. I had some pressure waves that would come and go, but nothing consistent. I woke up Friday morning, September 24th, and had some bloody show. I had an appointment with my OB and explained to her my symptoms. She checked me and I was 6 centimeters dilated and 90% effaced. My baby was at 0 station. She stripped my membranes and asked if I would like to go to the hospital that day. I told her I would rather go home and spend the day preparing for my little man's arrival.

I stayed busy all day cleaning and moving. My doula came and did some exercises with me to try to move things along. We had no luck. Saturday morning I woke up and I was miserable. I decided that afternoon that I wanted to go to the hospital, as I thought I had progressed further. When we got there, I was still 6 centimeters dilated. After 2 hours of working with the doula to try to speed things along, they sent us home. I was so uncomfortable and mentally and emotionally exhausted from the weeks of prodromal labor that I cried.

Sunday morning I decided to give the midwives brew a try around 10:00am. I then did some more exercises to help get my baby out. I also used my breast pump a few times to try and stimulate stronger contractions. The brew gave me some diarrhea but nothing too bad. I continued to bounce on my ball, do hip circles, and rest. I took a nap and then around 6:30pm I decided to do the miles circuit. I finished that around 8:00.

At 8:19pm I started having regular waves every 2-3 minutes lasting 30-45 seconds. They started out pretty strong and continued to intensify. I had my mom come get my daughter and called my doula to come back. She arrived by 9:30pm and as soon as she walked in, I had an intense wave and told her we needed to go. The car ride intensified the waves to the point that I was moaning very loudly through them. I told my partner that we needed to hurry because I was feeling the urge to push. When we walked into the ER at 10:02pm I was screaming. I couldn't find my focus or control my breathing. My doula kept trying to help me find my calm, but he was coming so fast. They rushed me to a room, took my pants off, and two roaring pushes later I had my baby in my arms at 10:06pm.

It was only 1 hour and 47 minutes from the time my contractions became consistent until my baby was out. I didn't get my calm collected hypnobabies birth that I envisioned, but I am so thrilled with how things turned out. It was intense and very uncomfortable but I didn't feel a "ring of fire." Everything happened so fast that I didn't get an IV and my doctor told them not to even worry about one. Baby latched on and nursed great. I had a small tear requiring a few stitches. We are both happy and healthy and I got my natural unmedicated birth.

Welcome to the world Beckham Grey. 7 pounds 14 ounces and 19.75 inches long.

September 28, 2021

Emi and Charlotte

I went into labor on September 27th at 41 weeks and 3 days pregnant via a hospital induction because I had developed preeclampsia. Due to this, I had to say goodbye to my home birth plans and try to make peace with the change. I asked for minimal interventions and no cervical checks, but was told I needed to have a cervical check to decide my method of induction. I often wonder if I had held my ground here and not agreed, perhaps my birth story would be a happy one. When I agreed, the doctor performed a membrane sweep without my consent. As a past sexual assault survivor it made it very hard to progress after that.

My labor was spent reliving traumas and in fight or flight mode. I was started on Pitocin and for the next 8 hours I had pain free, but incredibly productive contractions. When I had my next cervical check I was only 3 centimeters dilated. The doctor told me she "wanted me to be in pain," and turned the Pitocin up so high that after reaching insane levels of pain, my body gave out. It was not normal labor pain, or even Pitocin pain, but rather every nerve ending in my body screaming as my body was pushed past it's limits.

After that I had no choice but to get an epidural, which was ineffective, but came with a catheter. I was not warned of this beforehand, and catheters were one of my biggest fears. It got worse when the nurse blew the catheter up in my urethra and decided to put her hand in my vagina in order to push it into my bladder. After my epidural, I progressed quickly. I did not want my waters broken, but just before it was time to push the doctor told me she couldn't tell how dilated I was and had to break my waters. I so wish that informed consent had been a part of my birth experience and that I had been prepared for the scare tactics delivered.

It was like the doctors were purposely neglectful because I wasn't just doing whatever they wanted. When it came time to push, they forced me to push on my back, despite it being contraindicated due to a connective tissue disorder I have. I suffered a third degree tear. Out loud, they told me it was a first degree tear. It was only during the long and unfinished process of repairing the damage done at my birth that a new doctor verified that I did have a third degree tear.

After 27 minutes, my beautiful baby Charlotte Belladonna was born into this world. The event of her birth was one of the most horrifying and traumatizing days of my life due to the medical staff attending her birth, and I hope that I can tell my story to advocate for myself and all of the other mothers out there who are victims of obstetric violence. My daughter is the best part of my life, but I can never have her birth back.

September 30, 2021

Abi and Gatlin: A Birth in Virginia

I was such a happy pregnant person. I almost didn't want it to end! As I hit my due date, the messages came flooding in. "When's that baby coming?" or "Baby yet?" or "Why isn't he here yet?" My mentality was baby would come when he was ready. Eventually I got tired of getting the messages and decided to write a letter to my baby. I hoped that it would allow my body to feel ready and release any stress before going into labor. But there was still no sign of baby.

On September 29th I went to see my chiropractor for my routine visit. He was working on my round ligament and noticed that one side was just not letting up. I jokingly asked, "Does that mean I'm in labor?" He said, "Not necessarily, but not impossible!" I went about my day and went to work.

That evening my husband and I went to the grocery store to get some dinner. As the indecisive pregnant person, I settled with mozzarella sticks, french fries, and my classic ice cream with cereal on top. We finally got to bed around 10:30. I stayed up on my phone while my husband slept because I'm never ready to fall asleep when he is. I was laying in bed and felt a pop! My pelvis always popped when rolling over, so I didn't think much of it. I thought to myself I might as well go pee since I was still awake. When I stood up, I realized the pop was my water breaking.

My contractions started quickly but nothing felt unbearable. My midwife always said that if contractions start, try to sleep as much as possible while you are able to. I was not able to. Laying down felt like I was dying. Standing helped me flow through the contractions better, and I reminded myself to take each one at a time. My husband decided to call my midwife to keep her in the loop and she decided it was a good time for her to head towards us. I found myself running back and forth from my living room to my bathroom.

When my midwife and her team arrived, they did their routine checkups on me and baby. My contractions were heavy in my back and the only comfort I could find was sitting up leaning on my bed. My husband helped remind me to breathe and tried to comfort me through the contractions. The nausea was hitting me hard. I would think, "No, I'm not going to throw up..." and then run to the bathroom as fast as I could! I decided taking a shower would help pass some time and hopefully help ease my discomfort. After getting out, we thought it would be a good time to make our way downstairs towards the pool. Immediately after getting in, I felt the need to push.

In between contractions I admired the view outside on the foggy morning. While pushing on my hands and knees, it seemed like nothing was happening. I felt his head migrate down, but it wasn't progressing as fast as we had wanted it. After two hours of pushing in the tub, we all decided I needed to try something different. I tried pushing on the birthing stool, standing up with my knees pointed in, on my back, on my side. You name it, I tried it all! It seemed like we had hit a wall. I was pale, and my body was definitely getting exhausted.

My midwife encouraged me to try and pee, but no matter how hard I tried, nothing seemed to work. My whole team and my husband wanted me to get a catheter, but I did NOT want it. My husband was forcing ice cream down my throat when he looked at me and said, "It's either the catheter or we transfer." I got the catheter and had half of a quart sized mason jar of urine come out of my body! It was game on after that. Pushing on my back really allowed me to bear down and give as much as I could to every push. My baby was finally about to be here.

I needed to be patient as he crowned and used short breaths to get through the ring of fire. His head finally came out and a minute went by with no progress. My midwife's assistant said, "It's been a minute." They then looked at me and said I needed to flip to my hands and knees They helped me flip over. I felt so much pressure. I kept reminding myself it was almost over. I yelled hoping it would end soon. And then it was gone. The pressure released! My son needed some assistance, as he didn't come out breathing. After some patience, care, and love, my son Gatlin was finally here. The 12 hours of labor and 4 hours of pushing all felt worth it.

October

October 1, 2021

Nicole and Aubree: A Birth in Alberta, Canada

For the majority of my pregnancy, I was planning a hospital birth. Like many, I was sucked into the belief that "babies are born in a hospital." I genuinely thought home birth was just for hippies or for people that didn't make it to the hospital in time. My perspective changed as I began to learn more about how birth works and after realizing the amount of advocacy that would be required to have a natural birth in a hospital setting. I officially changed my mind and "committed" to preparing to have my baby at home part way through my third trimester.

Fast forward to 37 weeks. I had been experiencing mild period like cramping and losing parts of my mucous plug, but I was convinced that first time moms rarely have their baby early. I had been doing various things to prep my body for labour: eating dates, drinking red raspberry leaf tea, and seeing the chiropractor and acupuncturist. At exactly 38 weeks, after attending my regular acupuncture appointment, the cramping got more intense. I had been experiencing fairly strong Braxton Hicks contractions since about 26 weeks, so I was unsure if I'd be able to actually tell when I was in early labour. But these contractions felt different. They were also consistently 10 minutes apart.

I texted my doula to update her and she advised me to carry on with my day and not pay attention to them. I followed her guidance and took a warm bath and applied my TENS machine to my back before heading to bed. I went to sleep expecting the contractions to taper off. I woke up shortly before 2:00am, TENS machine still on. I'm not sure what woke me up, the contractions were still minor. I got up and went to the bathroom and noticed some bloody show. After this, my contractions quickly became more intense. After another text to my doula, her wise words came across my phone screen and read something like, "Stop timing your contractions. It's time to get out of your head and into your body. Animal brain turns on." I couldn't fall back to sleep and proceeded to labour alone around my house while my husband and dogs slept soundly.

I was weirdly calm and still in denial. I knew early labour could go on for a long time. Things continued to progress and around 6:00am I woke my husband up and suggested he not go to work that day. Within minutes of him contacting his boss, he suggested he time a few contractions, as he felt they were pretty close together. At this point I was still coping fairly well. I couldn't talk through contractions, and they would bring me down to my knees where I could confidently breathe through them. My husband timed a few and they were consistently 4-6 minutes apart.

Within half an hour, I was having a hard time simply "breathing through them." They were getting more intense, and we decided it was time to have our doula come. She arrived by 7:00am and quickly had me in positions that put gravity on my side. As the sun was rising and light began flooding the main floor of my house, she set up my bathroom with my affirmation cards and candles. I laboured on the toilet for quite awhile. I felt safe and secure. I knew my husband and doula were just on the other side of the door.

I began feeling nauseous and shaky around the same time my doula announced she was going to page my midwife. I had a feeling I was entering transition. My midwife arrived just before 10:00 and performed a cervical exam confirming I was 8-9 centimeters dilated. This was encouraging for me. I thought, "If I made it this far, I can do it!" Shortly after, I got into the birth pool that was set up in my living room. The warm water instantly helped my body to relax. Contractions were intense but I was feeling the most pain in my back. I now know I was experiencing back labour because baby was in the sunny side up position.

The back pain was by far the most uncomfortable part and I agreed to try sterile water injections. I think I got a bit of relief and continued to labour in the pool. Time felt slow and I remembered my water had not broken. A moment of panic ran through me and I worried that things were stalled because of my membranes remaining intact. My midwife said she could break them if I wanted her to, but warned me that it would likely cause things to become more intense. I didn't think I could handle more intense, so I declined. I remained in the pool for the rest of my labour. I began to feel the urge to push, so the second midwife was called.

Pushing felt very awkward for me, but with a bit of coaching, it was like a lightbulb went off and I understood how to coordinate my breath. I only pushed for 20 minutes before my daughter was born. As her head was crowning, she turned from sunny side up and my water broke while the second midwife was walking in the door.

Aubree Rae was born at 1:07pm on a sunny October afternoon. Moments after delivering her, my dogs greeted their new sister at the edge of the pool. My husband and I felt as if we'd known her forever. The room was calm, yet full of excitement. I birthed the placenta shortly after. I was worried when my midwife told me I'd have to push again, but relieved when she reminded me that placentas don't have bones. After cutting the cord, my husband held Aubree on his chest skin to skin while my midwives assisted me out of the pool. We enjoyed the golden hour in bed while the house got cleaned up. You'd never know I had a baby in my living room that day.

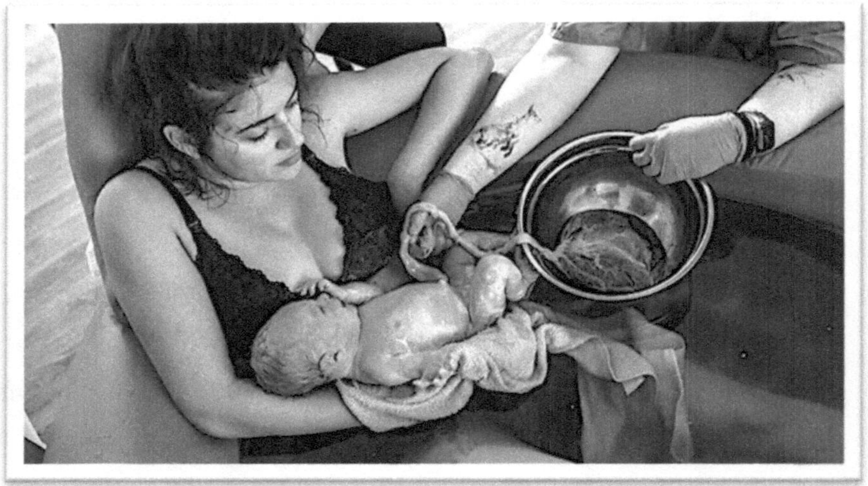

Photo by Lindsey
Adora Birth + Wellness

October 3, 2021

Abby and Millie

On Saturday October 2nd, I woke up feeling a little crampy with sporadic contractions. I had been having random contractions for a few weeks now, so I really didn't think this might be labor. However, my mindset was different. Instinctually I knew my baby was coming soon.

By noon the contractions were coming every 20 minutes and started to become closer together. Around dinner time they were 10-15 minutes apart, so I decided to let my midwife (who is also my mother in law!) know what was going on. My labors are typically very fast once I get into active labor, so we decided she would come over and bring her bags and equipment. Once she arrived, I asked her to check my cervix to see if these contractions were doing any work for us. She agreed and I was 2-3 centimeters dilated and 80% effaced. Knowing it was still early, she went back home and I got ready to go to bed.

I laid down around 9:00pm and the contractions ramped up. They were coming closer and stronger and I decided to get out of bed and go walk around. As I began to walk, I felt my body release a large gush of liquid. I yelled out to my husband that my water broke, and he immediately got up and started prepping the bed for birth time. I went to the bathroom to clean up. When I pulled down my pants, I noticed that the gush was actually blood and not amniotic fluid. I yelled for my husband to bring me my phone and called my midwife immediately. She rushed back over and assessed the blood loss. She said it was an amount she was comfortable with and guessed that it just meant our baby would be here soon.

My midwife suggested we listen to baby's heart rate and it was perfect. Shortly after I had another gush of blood. At this point my midwife did not think this was normal and asked to perform a vaginal exam again. During the exam I lost a large clot and more blood. She looked at my husband and said, "I need you to call 911." She explained that she suspected I was having a placental abruption and it was best I go to the hospital. A few minutes later, the ambulance arrived and off I went.

Once at the hospital, the OB agreed with my midwife that I was having a partial placental abruption. We quickly developed a game plan. If baby's heart rate stayed normal and I wasn't losing too much blood, I could continue to labor and have our baby naturally. I was thrilled, as many abruptions call for an immediate c-section. I continued to labor throughout the night and at 4:00am the OB came into the room. She said she was pleased with my blood loss and baby's heart rate but suggested a vaginal exam to see if there had been any progress. I agreed. I was 4 centimeters dilated. She started discussing augmentation since I hadn't progressed much in several hours. Her suggestions were Pitocin or breaking my bag of waters. I agreed to breaking my water.

A few minutes later I was contracting every couple of minutes, and they were very intense. Around 5:00am I looked at my husband and said, "The baby is coming down, I need you to go get the nurse." The nurse came in and asked to do another vaginal exam, in which she found I was complete. She called for the doctor as I began bearing down. The doctor walked in the room and I began pushing. In 2 short pushes I felt my baby begin to emerge. She had a nuchal cord, so the doctor unwrapped it. At 5:08am, I reached down and pulled Millie up to my chest.

We spent an hour skin to skin and she latched on to breastfeed very quickly. There were no further complications from the abruption or my blood loss. A hospital transfer may sound like a homebirthers worst nightmare, but I am thrilled and grateful we have a medical system to help care for us if an emergency arises.

October 4, 2021

Erica and Jeanie

I knew after two hospital births that this pregnancy was going to be different. I was ready to take complete control of my body and my pregnancy. I also knew the way to do that was by planning for a home birth. I found an amazing and supportive midwife and team, and they let me call all of the shots.

On October 4th I woke up with contractions about five minutes apart. I got in the bath around 10:00am and decided that was where I was going to stay for a while. My sweet sister told me that my contractions were about 2-3 minutes apart. I was sure there was no way I was close to birth, because I was so at peace and almost blissful in the bath. I even told my husband to go and get us coffee because it would be a while!

At 10:50 I got out of the bath and had to crawl to my bed. Little did I know I was in transition. My midwife called and I told her that I was fine! My contractions were now a minute apart and I did not want any stimulation. No music, no lights, no touching... nothing. I was talking to my daughter, letting her know that we were safe. I looked at my husband, told him I wasn't scared, but my water was going to break and "It's about to get real." He very nicely and sternly told me I needed to change positions from laying on my side once my water broke so gravity could do it's job.

It was just me, my sister, and my husband at home. As soon as I got on all fours, a noise came from my stomach to my throat and out of my mouth that I had never heard before. With that scream my body started to push. I felt her head. I told my husband to fill up the birth tub, but by the time he turned around to grab the hose I yelled, "She's coming out!" When he turned around I was holding our sweet Baby Jeanie. It was 11:27am. Fetal election reflex is amazing. She came flying out like a damn football. I caught her with one hand all by myself. It was amazing. Life changing. Magic. I will forever love my body more because of what she did that day.

October 9, 2021

Monet and Hilux

After 41 weeks and 2 days, I got to meet my beautiful baby boy. He came into this world in the most natural way and grew in the most natural way with no medical intervention or ultrasounds. Welcome to the world my Hilux Blu.

Prodromal labor began the night of October 6th and lasted through the night, waking me continuously. I brushed these contractions off as Braxton Hicks, but they continued on and off through the day of the 7th and continuously woke me throughout that night. They continued through the day of the 8th to the point I was in so much pain, I laid in the bath and cried from the pain and lack of sleep. I began keeping track of my contractions, and around 7:00pm on the 8th I realized they were roughly 5 minutes apart and early labor was beginning.

Taylor filled my birthing pool and began to set everything up. I called my mom and friends to come by and witness the birth of my baby. Labor continued, I screamed, cried, and roared, but did not progress. I stayed at 3 centimeters for roughly 6 hours. I was delusional from lack of sleep and an inability to calm myself enough to take a deep breath. I cried thinking my body was failing me and I wouldn't be able to have the natural birth I dreamed of. I completely discredited my body. I thought I wasn't progressing and would need to take something to get my baby out. I thought I would need a c-section because my body wasn't capable of birth. But then I remembered the affirmations and breathing techniques I had practiced for the last nine months while I was pregnant.

I began to chant, "Open up!" with each contraction and would speak words of encouragement to myself like, "I am elastic" and "I'm going to meet my baby!" Within the hour I went from being stuck at 3 centimeters to feeling the fetal ejection reflex kick in. My body was beginning to push. I was in disbelief until I reached down and felt my babies head, still intact in the amniotic sac.

I continued to scream and roar and yell, with each contraction pushing my baby lower and lower. I held my mom's hands though each contraction, the generations of love. Taylor was behind me in the pool rubbing my back and keeping an eye on the baby, ready to catch them. I felt the head come out and go back in many times while pushing. Finally, Taylor saw the amniotic sac burst when our babies head was almost all the way out.

I continued to let the fetal ejection reflex do its job and get my baby out while I continued to scream and remind myself that I would meet my baby soon. It was almost over. All this pain was for a reason, and that reason was almost in my arms. All of a sudden, my baby was born! He slid right out and into his father's arms. Taylor lifted our baby out of the water where he instantly began to cry. I turned around and Taylor placed him on my chest and then exclaimed, "It's a boy!"

Taylor and I cried, looking at each other and our new baby with more love than I can even describe.

I did it! I birthed my baby! All naturally at home in a pool, the way nature intended. The way I dreamed of. Everything progressed when I began to trust my body. It was me holding my baby back. On October 9th, at 3:03am, the love of my life Hilux Blu was born into his father's arms. He weighed 8 pounds and 1 ounce. The most perfect baby I've ever seen.

October 13, 2021

Lauren and Blake

My home birth was a surprisingly healing experience for me. When I was pregnant with my first baby, I had planned to have an unmedicated birth. I spent months practicing hypnobirthing, visualizing, and receiving care from the midwives at my local hospital. I ended up having an intervention-heavy induction and vacuum assisted delivery. Having had such a wild turn of events with my first, my birth desires for my second baby were less clear to me.

During my second pregnancy we relocated to a different state. The closest hospital that offered the model of care I was used to was 50 minutes away. There were plenty of hospitals closer, but I didn't feel like they would be a good fit for me. With every prenatal appointment my anxiety grew. The drive was SO FAR. What if I didn't make it in time? Covid precautions were still in place and I knew they weren't going to allow my then 21 month old to join us in the hospital. I had not been away from my child for more than a few hours her whole life. The thought of being away from her during such a sensitive time broke my heart.

At 37 weeks, I called my doula and asked if she knew how I could go about having my baby at home. She connected me with the midwives that had delivered her baby! In that moment, the most perfect birthing team was formed. These women provided my final weeks of prenatal care, and at 41 weeks and 5 days, they came over to assist me with the birth of my baby in the middle of the night. It was wild and glorious and so much messier than I could have ever imagined. I remember reciting my affirmations one minute and babbling on about needing an epidural the next minute. I remember feeling so incredibly calm and capable during one surge and yelling "Help me!" during the next. It didn't look or feel anything like the beautiful birth photography I had poured over for years and the thought of that kept making me laugh on the inside.

Right before transition I experienced the most peaceful rest. My midwife had just given me IV fluids and we played a hypnobirthing track. I immediately got back into a state of calm. My husband said everyone became silent and rested with me until I was ready to deliver. Something much greater than me took over after that rest and I stood up and walked over to the bathtub. I gave birth to my son in the water. In that moment I felt simultaneously out of body and more present with myself than I'd ever been. He was perfectly healthy and weighed 9 pounds and 1 ounce. Although I had experienced a third-degree tear with my first baby, this time I stayed completely intact. In the comfort of my home, with an experienced team of birth workers, I felt so safe and cared for the entire time. Having my husband and daughter join the new baby and me in bed immediately after was the best feeling.

October 14, 2021

Miarra and Olivia

It started around 1:30am. I called Heidi and Beverly, my midwives, around 2:00am. Then we called Molly, our birth photographer. Contractions started to get more intense around 5:00am and I wanted to go in my room alone. I paced back and forth, listening to birth affirmations from a hypnobirthing app. Around 7:00 I was ready to say screw it and just send everyone home since my contractions were steady but not getting closer together. That's when I told my husband that we should go for a walk. I was ready for bed and tired of pacing back and forth in my home. We made it to the mailbox at the end of our driveway when it felt like a water balloon popped in my stomach and I screamed, "Ohh F***! I ain't going nowhere." Molly and Kenneth chuckled. They thought I was joking. I said it again. "No, I'm not going anywhere. She's about to come now. My water just broke."

That's when shit got real. We came back inside and told the midwives and I got in the birth pool at 7:35am. I would say I had about 8-10 contractions in the birth pool all together. They almost took me out. I kept asking for ice and water and then the puke bucket. The whole time my husband was rubbing my back and holding me up, repeatedly saying, "You're doing a great job baby. Breathe baby." I remember the ninth contraction in the pool. I groaned and put my hand down and felt a face and hair. I prayed, "Jesus help me, I can do this, I just need your help."

One knee was down and the other leg was in a lunge. My body felt good in that position. The midwives said, "Whenever you're ready, you can grab her body out." Olivia's head stayed under water for about 45 seconds and then the next contraction came. One big push and I reached and pulled and she was out at 8:23am. After I caught my baby, I caught my breath. We walked to my comfy king size bed and took a nap with my placenta lying next to me and Olivia still attached to it. After we rested, she was weighed. She weighed 7 pounds and 10 ounces and was 19 inches long.

Welcome to the world Olivia Grace.

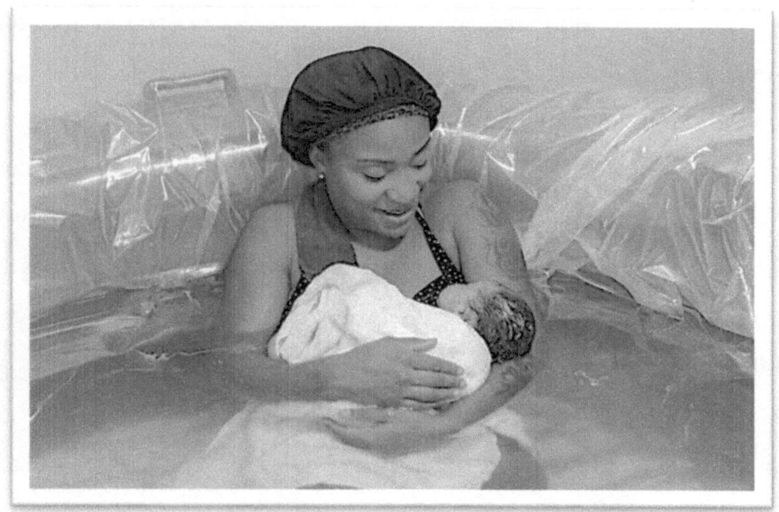

Photo by Molly Blunier
Molly Blunier Photography

October 14, 2021

Abigail and Yves

I woke up a bit after 4:00am with light contractions. I laid in bed and felt so happy — I had waited 41 weeks for my baby's birthday. I had endured abdominal surgery and a cancer scare. I had also weighed the risks of another possible placental abruption with both my midwife and a seemingly endless team of gynecologists.

The surges continued and with them my confidence in my body grew. The doubts I had following my induction for Julian's birth washed away. My body knew how to go into labor!

I woke up Joe and he timed contractions for a bit, then we got up. I focused on relaxing during the surges and got ready for the day in between. Julian got up at 5:30, which worked out beautifully, as he could keep to his routine and have breakfast and get ready for the day with Joe.

Joe called my doula and my midwife at 6:00am. He helped get my mom and Julian sorted, then turned his attention to me. I could have done it without Joe, but I thrived with his support. He protected my bubble, he whispered affirmations and visualizations to help me relax, he physically supported me as I surrendered to the process of birth.

Our doula arrived around 7:00, and my midwife around 8:00. They prepared things and set up the birthing tub while I was tucked away in my bubble. I had one brief interruption to listen to baby's heartbeat. I got in the tub around 9:30 — a soothing reward that allowed for freedom of movement and eased the pressure. It also slowed my contractions. When I felt the need to press, I surrendered. I filled my belly with air to give my baby space to move and squatted as my body told me to. I focused on relaxing my body, shaking out my hands when necessary and sending my energy downward.

His head was born still in the sac, and I swayed in the water, waiting another two minutes for the next contraction. I trusted he was safe. I trusted in the reflex to breathe not yet being triggered. I trusted in the process of birth. I trusted in the placenta and umbilical cord to keep him safe.

Just before 11:00am, he was born into the water, and I lifted him to my chest. I peeled back a veil of amniotic sac that remained on his sweet head. Yves' birth was everything I dreamed of and desired. I felt neither fear nor doubt. It answered lingering questions I had since Julian's birth about my body's ability to labor naturally, and about my own power.

It was the kind of birth people don't talk about, but they should. No drama, no emergency, no screaming. A normal, uncomplicated, peaceful birth.

October 21, 2021

Lydia and Jedrek: A Birth in Ontario, Canada

I had some serious Braxton Hicks for weeks prior to my son's birth. It was challenging mentally, emotionally, and physically, but it was all preparing my body for birth. The morning of October 20th I lost my mucus plug at 11:30am and was had some strong cramping. I had been in touch with my doula for weeks at this point because of how often I thought I was in labour, but that day my hopes weren't high. I was focused on intentionally connecting with Calla and we made play dough for the first time. I had a midwife appointment at 2:30 that I didn't want to go to, but I did anyway. It was good to get out of the house.

The contractions were very inconsistent up until this point. I had read somewhere that pumping can help increase contractions. Pumping releases oxytocin, which is what signals your uterus to contract. I knew about pumping but never felt the need to do it until after my midwife appointment. There was this thing in me that kept telling me to go relax and pump for 10 minutes. I listened to it, and my contractions got intense for the next couple hours.

Things slowed down around 5:30pm, which was nice. I got Calla to bed and relaxed with Johnny for a bit. The contractions picked up again and so I pumped again for 10 minutes to see what would happen. Usually at night the contractions would start around 5:00, go till about 9:00, and then just stop. This time they felt different. After I pumped the contractions really amped up with consistency and strength. I tried to get some sleep, but it wasn't happening.

The contractions were manageable, but I had to focus on my breathing. I kept in contact with Rianne, my doula, the whole time with how I was doing and feeling. I still thought this wasn't the real deal. At 11:00pm I had the most intense contraction yet. My instinct was to tense up and fight it. I did that but then gathered myself and came back to a relaxed state. Fear. Tension. Pain. If we stop the fear, we decrease tension, and then the pain is very minimal or nonexistent. Rianne was on her way, Johnny got up and went and slept downstairs, and I was having a baby!

Rianne got here around 11:30 and her presence was so peaceful. Her touch was calming and her help was so needed. I labored with my knees on the floor while I leaned over the bed. I felt I could move best with my contractions this way. Rianne oiled me up and did heat on my back while applying counter pressure on my tailbone, where I felt every contraction. She kept offering me water and made sure I stayed hydrated. It was that one contraction that hit when I said, "I need to poop."

I moved super slowly to the bathroom and sat on the toilet for a long time. The contractions got intense. Baby was coming! I stayed on the toilet for a while and then started feeling the urge to push. This whole time I was checking myself. I wasn't feeling for how dilated I was, but for gauging where Jedrek was sitting. I could feel his head after a couple of pushes and it was so exciting.

With Jedrek getting so close to coming, my body was making room by puking, peeing and pooping. If I'm being honest with you, I love puking while in labor. I wanted to puke when Calla was born, and when I started to feel the urge with Jedrek it was actually a relief. It made the contractions way less intense. By 1:00am Rianne was like, "Hey girl, we should probably call the midwives, you are getting really close." I didn't think so because of how long I labored with Calla, but she assured me it wouldn't be long and the midwives needed time to get here. We chatted about catching him, just me and her (I secretly wish that happened, wouldn't that have been a story to tell.)

We waited another 15 minutes and then called the midwives. I loved both of my midwives very much, but I knew the one from Calla's birth best and I loved her energy she brought to the room. Calm. Peaceful. Gentle. Understanding. I was lucky that she was the one coming to my birth again! While I was waiting for Kim to get here, I started to realize my body was doing a lot of pushing but not moving the baby. I was becoming tired. I again listened to my body, and it was asking for a shower, so we did that. Oh my, that felt good!

The contractions flowed away with the water. Literally. They slowed down and allowed me to have more rest in between. I was so exhausted and so ready to be done. I really wanted it over already, but the slow down of contractions was exactly what I needed even if it wasn't what I wanted. I was able to recollect myself and nap a tad. There was a shift in the contractions once they came back. I found that letting my body shake them off was working best. I don't know how to describe it. I was on my hands and knees in the shower. I pushed against the shower seats to provide counter pressure. I lost Jedrek's head, I couldn't feel it anymore. I cried. I felt like labor was never going to end.

I felt like I wouldn't meet my little boy. I loved having Rianne there to support me when I was feeling defeated like this. She's seriously the best. As the contractions got stronger again, I got extremely tired. I wasn't staying focused and was spiraling to a dangerous head space. I hadn't eaten since supper, so I needed some fuel. Thank goodness for Ningxia because it gave me liquid energy. I still wasn't keeping a lot down, but the Ningxia was working. I was feeling energized and ready to get this baby out. After a few really good, deep contractions and I felt his head again. WE GOT THIS!

He came down really quickly again and was sitting on one bone just like Calla had. I knew what to do. I helped him move down with a couple assisted pushes. I don't mean hold your breath and go blue in the face pushes. It's like pulling your abs in nice and tight and pushing their bums down. After a couple of those and he was good.

While doing all this Kim arrived and set up her supplies while letting me do my thing. She so sweetly asked if I wanted her in the room or out and I so unsweetly responded, "If you're quiet, you can stay. So shhhh." I really liked my zone and bubble of me and Rianne. It was everything I needed and wanted. My water broke as soon as he passed that pelvic bone and then he was crowing. It was a LOT of pressure. I held his head for the last couple contractions to let things stretch and avoid tearing. Then his head was out. I've never experienced the ring of fire people talk about. After a couple more contractions, he was in my arms.

He didn't cry, but that's not a bad thing. Not all baby's need to cry. He was cozy hanging out on my chest, nice and warm. I had an awesome birth. My post birth was so much better this time. I was chatty and felt amazing. When it was time to birth the placenta, Kim pulled out a bottle of Clary Sage and just opened it and my body was ready to let go. My placenta slid right out. No pulling, no touching.

After a while Kim asked, "Do you want to cut the cord soon?" I was in my birth high and asked, "Are you rushing me, or has it been a good amount of time?" It had been over 30 minutes since Jedrek was born. I was just making sure he got everything he needed from the placenta before cutting the cord. This whole labor was hands off and amazing. Rianne got to cut the cord. It's not my thing and I love that she got to do that for me. I showered and got all cozy in bed, Josh came and I got to sleep while he was watching Jedrek. What once was the unknown is life today.

October 22, 2021

Krystle and Bear: A Birth in England

After already having three large natural birth babies, I was told my fourth would most likely be even bigger, and especially because it was a boy this time round. I had growth scans during the pregnancy and on the final growth scan, two weeks before my due date, the sonographer stated my baby was very large and weighed approximately 10 pounds and 7 ounces. The doctor made a fuss and stated that they thought scheduling a cesarean would be the safest option for my birth. I was informed that if I went into labour naturally,

I must attend the hospital immediately, as they didn't want the baby to start coming and his shoulders get stuck. I felt shocked by what the doctor said. I never wanted a cesarean and I didn't want to be cut open.

That night I was woken at 4:45am by my 2-year-old and realized that my water had broken. My partner rushed me to the hospital where I was given another scan to check the size and position of the baby. I was informed yet again that the baby was huge.

I never experienced any contractions, just a few mild tightenings while awaiting to go into theatre. On entering theatre, I felt terrified, as I didn't know what to expect. I was frightened by the drips being placed into both my hands and then wondered what was going to happen to me once the doctor had finished injecting a spinal into my lower back, which hurt. I continued to remain silent, just watching and listening to everything that was happening around me and to me.

I laid down on the operating table and within a few short minutes my son was being held up above the curtain that was covering me. I was so pleased to see him. I couldn't believe how quickly they had got him out.

I cried as I was so pleased that he was here safe and well. I then heard the midwife state, "He's not 10 pounds, he's not even 9 pounds..." She then weighed him with my partner and he weighed 8 pounds and 8 ounces. The doctors said to me, "You could have sneezed him out!" and laughed. My previous baby that I had birthed naturally was over 10 pounds, so there really had been no need for the cesarean. I was only given a cesarean due to the predicted size of my baby.

All I can remember thinking to myself whilst still lying on the operating table was, "I don't care what he weighs as long as he is healthy. My beautiful son, Bear William Ragnar."

October 23, 2021

Gabriele and Ellison

Waking up to the sounds of little feet chasing each other is the perfect beginning to every Saturday morning. I rolled out of bed filled with joy and energy, which was an odd feeling for being 41 weeks pregnant. The house was prepared to welcome a baby into and our home-birth plan was waiting to be executed. After having one medicated hospital birth and two unmedicated hospital births, this was new territory for us. But we were eager to watch it all unfold. My husband and I decided we were going to spend the day spoiling our three girls before we welcomed their new sister.

We all got ready and loaded into the car to go to a local doughnut shop. Traffic was quite terrible and I was feeling car sick, so we opted to change the plans and grab some doughnuts from the grocery store closer to home. We arrived back home and the car sicknesses didn't subside. We texted our holistic doula and told her that we thought I was in the beginning stages of labor, and we would play the day by ear. I decided that I wanted to take one last uninterrupted shower before welcoming another sweet baby. We called a friend to pick up the older kids. I hopped in to enjoy one nice hot shower and realized I was progressing a lot faster than I thought I was earlier. I wasn't worried though because my doula was on her way and my husband was…wait where was my husband? Mopping the floor! I mean what else would a husband who is nervously waiting on his fourth daughter be doing?

I was an hour into what we thought was just car sickness and I was definitely in active labor. I felt the most peaceful in our master bedroom, so I had set it up to be a calming environment. I had every fan in the house going, but it was just not enough. I needed a cup of ice and my husband notified me that we had none. But I NEEDED it. He decided that he would listen to that gentle command and went to the store just 5 minutes away from home. I heard the front door open, and it was the doula and my husband. I was at the point of focused labor and she could tell. She jumped right in and could see that the position I was in was not helping the baby descend.

I changed into a few different positions and my doula actively applied counter pressure through contractions. She notified me that my water broke and reminded me that I wanted to birth in the water. My husband got the bath ready for us and we transitioned to the bathtub for a water birth. Once I was in the water, I could tell that baby was going to make her appearance. My husband patiently waited and caught baby a short two pushes later. We wept tears of joy. Ellison Vera was welcomed into this world two hours after the onset of labor and immediately was wrapped up into the hands of her loving father who transferred her to the arms of her loving mother.

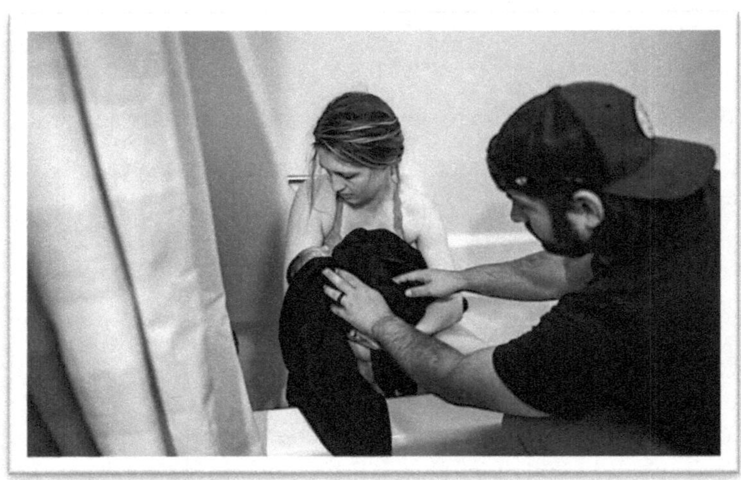

October 24, 2021

Lauren and Hugh

On Sunday morning I started to feel the start of my contractions but didn't think anything of them. As the day progressed, I felt the surges become more consistent and intense. At 4:00pm, my husband arrived home from work and I told him, "Today is the day we get to meet our second baby." We both finished packing our hospital bags and spent our last moments with our son as a family of three. After my eldest child went to bed, so did my partner. We didn't know how long we would be waiting to meet our second born.

As the hours went by, the intensity of the surges became stronger and they moved closer together. Then my water broke at 7:00pm. By 8:00 my mucous plug had dislodged and I notified the midwives at the hospital that I would be arriving later that night. My contractions were approximately 4 minutes apart and lasting for 30-40 seconds.

While Daniel was sleeping, I was plotting around the house, doing the laundry, and making sure everything was clean. I find cleaning relaxing and satisfying. This was my personal technique of dealing with the discomfort. At 9:00pm the midwives contacted me to see how I was doing. The contractions had become closer, but also sporadic. The midwives asked if I would go in to be monitored. I told them I would like to wait another hour and see how I progress.

At 9:45pm, I rang my parents to come over so they could be there for William while we were away. I woke Daniel up and let him know we needed to leave soon. At 10:15 my parents arrived, and I remember my Dad asking me how far apart me contractions were. At this stage, my surges were 1 minute and 20 seconds apart and lasting 45-60 seconds.

We arrived at the hospital at 11:10pm and our allocated midwife is one women in my life I will never forget! She turned the lights down as soon as we entered the room and she didn't do a vaginal examination. Then she quickly read over my clinical notes. Daniel got out the music, bosu ball, gym mats, and applied acupressure whenever I was contracting. The acupressure was amazing! The bosu ball was what got me through the surges, rocking back and forth and bouncing.

After a while, I requested a vaginal exam, as I wanted to know how dilated I was. The midwife double checked I wanted to know and told me I was 8 centimeters. At this point the on-call obstetrician walked in and briefly introduced himself.

After the examination, I needed to go to the toilet. When I stood up I felt my baby drop into my pelvic floor. I went into the bathroom and tried to sit on the toilet and couldn't sit because of how heavy my pelvic floor felt. I walked back out into the birthing suite and told my midwife.

The midwife asked if I wanted to go in the shower, so I walked into the bathroom, stripped down without a care, and I remember thinking, "Gosh, I must be in transition, because I really don't care that I'm stark naked right now, on all fours." The warm water was on my lower back and Daniel continued the acupressure. Then I heard a voice behind me say, "We need to turn the water off and put some towels down." So I maneuvered myself around so that my head was facing the wall and my rear end was facing toward the voice.

I didn't know that Daniel had left the bathroom to have the conversation of "No medical interventions without giving us the pros and cons first." Daniel was in the hallway introducing himself to the obstetrician when the midwife called out to them, "The babies head is out!" They both walked into the bathroom and saw the midwife holding my little one.

From my perspective, I started roaring when I knew the head was coming out. My body pushed the baby out on its own. The head came out in two contractions, then they stopped. This is when my body had a rest and I felt the baby turn inside of me. After a long pause between surges, my body did one more push and my baby arrived.

The midwife passed him to me between my legs and Daniel told me we had another boy. As I picked him up, I could not have been more proud of what the two of us had accomplished. We did it together. Then I got up and walked to the bed in the birthing suite.

The umbilical cord was not clamped until the pulsating stopped and the whiteness appeared. Then it was cut by Daniel. I birthed the placenta naturally. The midwife explained the placenta and how the baby sits and grows within the amniotic sac. It was so amazing!

I had a one-degree tear, which didn't require stitches.

Hugh was born at 11:54pm.

Later on, the midwife told me I was actually 10 centimeters when she did the examination, not 8!

October 25, 2021

Jalina and Adler

My husband, Anthony, and I planned for a freebirth of our fourth baby in the last week of October 2021. On the evening of Monday, October 25th, I heard our 19-month-old fall and begin to cry. I hurried to squat down and hug him and felt a pop. My water poured into a puddle at the bottom of the stairs at 5:57pm. Anthony started an early bedtime for our three oldest children. The little ones walked through my amniotic fluid puddle on their way to bed, and I continued to leak at the bottom of the stairs until deciding at 7:22pm that I'd rather leak in the shower.

I took my time enjoying my shower before feeling my first painless contraction at 8:44pm. The next contraction came 10 minutes later. At 9:00, I was still leaking water. Contractions were mild and steadily increased in frequency from 10 minutes apart to about 3 minutes apart over the next 1.5 hours. During that time, I relaxed on my knees over some towels on our Nugget play couch. Finally, the leaking slowed. I alternated bouncing on the birth ball and walking around the living room, enjoying a snack platter and watching The Voice with Anthony.

At 10:23pm, I felt the first intense contraction and retreated into a quiet, softly lit room. Knowing labor could last all night, I rested on my side on our Nugget couch with a pillow between my legs. A contraction came that I really had to work through, so I had Anthony apply pressure to my sacrum. It did offer some relief, but after a second intense contraction that had me feeling stuck and punching the wall, I had to get up.

With each contraction, Anthony would hold my hand and sway side to side with me, rubbing my lower back. I would rub my belly gently and talk to my baby. We worked through a few contractions that way until I began feeling like I didn't want to go through many more.

I felt like I wanted to puke. I didn't exactly feel nauseated, but I thought puking might offer some sort of relief from the intense pressure concentrated on my cervix. At that point, I felt both logically and intuitively that I needed to get into a position that would open my pelvis. We had three Nugget mats stacked against the wall and one on the floor in front of that, so I got on my knees with my elbows up on the stacked mats and my feet spread apart.

Contractions became really intense, and I didn't know what to do to get relief. "Everything sucks," I said between contractions that were now coming every 2-3 minutes. I felt like I was wimping out after such a short time in labor. I recognized these feelings as signs of transition but didn't believe I could possibly be that close already. I had Anthony get me some ice water and start my birth playlist.

I made my way onto hands and knees but became tired from holding myself up. Anthony brought me the birth ball to lean on so I could relax my body and surrender to the contractions. I pep-talked and moaned my way through each one. Soon, the moans morphed into grunts. I was experiencing FER and could feel the baby coming down through the birth canal!

Finally, I felt the first ring of fire. With each ring of fire, I would regain control from the FER and tell myself, "Relax. Breathe. Stretch." I did this four times until the head was born. After the head was born, my contractions stopped. I wiggled my hips back and forth to allow my body to stretch and encourage another contraction. Anthony said calmly and firmly from behind me, "I need you to push." I trusted him. I practiced 3 gentle pushes to figure out what muscles to use, and the baby was born with the fourth push at 11:18pm.

After a couple minutes of helping the baby transition, Anthony helped me onto my back and handed me our fourth son. I held him close to my chest and cried out, "My baby! Thank you, God!" He was here, crying and flailing in my hands after being inside me just moments earlier. I was in utter disbelief.

The placenta came out easily 15 minutes later. Anthony cut the cord, helped me get comfortable, and began cleaning up. We ate, encouraged the baby to latch, discussed middle names, and processed the birth before finally going to bed around 4:00am. We weighed and measured the baby over the next couple days. It was so nice not being on someone else's schedule to do these things. We will undoubtedly plan to freebirth any future children.

October 26, 2021

Brooke and Kiah: A Birth in North Dakota

I woke up on the morning of October 26th at 3:55am with mixed emotions. Five minutes after waking up, I called the birthing center to make sure there was a bed available like I was told to do. Indeed, they were all ready for my 5:00am induction.

My mixed emotions included dread, fear, excitement, and sadness. Dread because I had heard too many stories of women being induced and the process taking over 24 hours. Fear because my firstborn, Jaxon, came on his own eight days late. I had an idea of labor and birth, but I did not know how the process of being induced worked. Excitement because the idea of meeting our baby was becoming real! Sadness because I was feeling as though my body had failed me by not going into labor naturally after all the miles of walking, gallons of raspberry tea I had drank, and every other tip and trick I had tried. I was also heart-broken because my midwife was not able to attend my birth after she chose not to be vaccinated. This was not my choice, but the hospitals. I had found out at my 39 week checkup that she was no longer allowed to have contact with her patients.

I arrived at the birthing center at 5:00am, changed into the gown, and went into the bed. Once they started the induction process, I felt my first contraction at 7:32am. The contraction was enough to notice, but nothing unbearable. It was much different than my labor with Jaxon where I did not feel any contractions until the middle of the night and I could no longer sleep through them.

My husband fell back asleep once we arrived at the birthing center. I watched tv, texted my sister to keep her updated, texted my best friend who had been induced three months early, and simply just tried to take in the day.

It was about 11:30 when Pitocin was first administered. Dr. T. was not lying when she said the contractions would worsen. They certainly hit different. The nurse kept encouraging an epidural. I am not against epidurals, but I delivered Jaxon without one and wanted to try to do so again.

Pretty soon I was unable to stay awake between contractions. Though the sleep was only a few minutes at a time, it was some of the very best sleep of my life! My nurse knew I was trying to last as long as I could without an epidural, but she had the anesthesiologist come in and talk me through the process just in case I were to change my mind. I could barely stay awake through his spiel, but he got through it, and I was relieved when he left and I didn't have to force myself to stay awake any longer.

Right about 3:00pm, Dr. T came back to break my water. "I'll be back at 5:15 after the clinic closes to come check on you if nothing happens beforehand!" I dreaded the thought of another two hours of this labor. Jaxon was born five hours after I arrived at the hospital. I was now going on ten hours at the hospital and still no baby.

About 10 minutes after breaking my water, I could no longer handle the contractions. I told the nurse I wanted the epidural. As she was walking out of the room to find the anesthesiologist, there was a total shift in my body! "WAIT, I NEED TO PUSH!" The nurse came running back and checked me. She was now on a mission to find Dr. T and the pediatric nurse. The peds nurse came right away, but Dr. T was not coming.

When I was first introduced to Dr. T at my 36 week checkup, she was a half hour late to the appointment. Once again, Dr. T took a half hour to show up when I needed her. I had to hold my baby in for ten contractions as I waited for her to arrive. Once she did show up, all it took was one contraction and five minutes of pushing for our little girl to arrive at 3:54pm.

This was not the birth I expected between my midwife being fired, being induced, and holding my baby in for way too many contractions. However, Kiah bear is the most perfect little girl I could ever hold in my arms and I would go through the whole process over again for her!

October 28, 2021

Elisha and Gianni: A Breech Birth in California

My birth story begins the night before my due date as I sat very pregnant on my living room floor. My sweet Labrador, Lucy, was very affectionate, following me all around the house and then finally nestling in between my legs with her head on my belly as I sat on the floor. Dogs have amazing instincts and that night I started the process of my "bloody show" although with no contractions.

This was my second baby and he decided at 33 weeks to settle in the breech position. I was lucky enough to already be in the prenatal care of the incredible Dr. Stuart Fischbein who specializes in breech, twins and VBAC home births. He had delivered my first son who was a head-down baby at home and I adore him. He quelled my fears of a natural breech birth with videos and information on the process.

270

Breech births are truly another version of normal and the technique for breech deliveries is unfortunately becoming a lost art to the profitable c-sections. I realized that this was the way my son wanted to be born. It was his choice, so why shouldn't I honor that choice? We were both healthy, so I was ready for the new experience.

After the bloody show began, it stopped as fast as it had started-leaving me in complete mystery. Two days later I started very sporadic contractions that lasted during the morning, then stopped, they began again in the evening, then stopped. I went to bed and contractions started again, then they stopped and then nothing! Over a period of 3 days, my body was slowly but surely dilating and preparing for the birth of this beautiful baby. Although frustrating to me, my body knew exactly what it was doing and therefore, made the laboring process much easier. I was able to sleep, drink, eat and relax over the course of those days. It really made me trust my body and trust the process.

Finally, a day came when I spent half a night having sporadic contractions and being on FaceTime with my amazing virtual doula, Krisha Crosley. My wonderful husband and I worked for three hours doing various poses during contractions to encourage the baby to descend into the right position before everything stopped once again. It was like the quiet before a storm! I had a 9:00am visit from my great midwife, Hayley Oakes, and was happy to learn that my cervix was very soft and I was around 5-6 centimeters dilated. With very few contractions, I took it easy that morning and did a few more relaxing poses to encourage my body and baby to continue the process of labor.

Around lunchtime that Thursday afternoon, my mom, who was taking care of my other son during this intense week, came for a visit and smoothie delivery. We visited for a bit just chatting in the kitchen about the excitement over the pending arrival, when I had a strong urge to use the restroom. I ran in there just fast enough for my water to break into the toilet. We immediately called Dr. Stu. After showing him a picture of the water, he knew this meant the time had come! He was seeing patients, so excused himself and jumped into his car as he was 40 minutes away from my house.

Luckily, my midwife was only 20 minutes away. Once my water broke, the contractions came on so fast and so intense that my husband was getting ready to catch the baby if needed! I was still on the toilet and felt the intense urge to push, so my doula quickly had me get off and onto all fours on the bed. The contractions were now coming so fast and so intense with the help of gravity, that it definitely was a most profound and powerful moment for me. I never doubted once in my mind that I couldn't do it, but I had to dig down deep and use all my strength and energy to accomplish this amazing feat. With the doctor on speaker, driving and assisting the midwife, I labored on. He got to our house and was there for 18 minutes before my sweet son arrived. He descended butt first, legs popped down, then arms and head.

I reached through my legs as the doctor handed me this little floppy body. With big wondering eyes, my son looked up at me as I hugged him close. My husband was by my side the whole time with encouraging words. He was my rock through it all. I held my baby feeling the power of a woman with this beautiful gift of life we have the honor to house and give forth. The breech birth was as incredible, beautiful and natural as nature intended it to be. I am so grateful and thankful that I got to experience both births of my sons in the beautiful calm setting of my home. Their births were different yet so similar.

I hope by sharing my story it can shine a light on the beauty and normalcy of a natural breech delivery.

<h1 style="text-align:center">November</h1>

November 1, 2021

Leah and Indie

Indie was born on Monday, November 1st at 4:32am. Her estimated due date was October 31st.

I woke up as if it were any other Sunday morning. It was a beautiful crisp fall day in Katonah. My two older daughters were up and about. Like most Sundays, we planned to make breakfast together. But this wasn't just any Sunday morning, it was HALLOWEEN! The girls were excited for the day and their candy-fueled evening.

When I went to the bathroom around 8:00am I noticed a lot of mucous in my underwear. I immediately wondered if it was my mucous plug. I mentioned it to my husband and went about the day with the girls. About an hour later I started to feel a gentle trickle of water run down my leg. I didn't think too much of this, but I did go to the bathroom to "investigate" and had more trickle. I told my husband I thought my water had broken so we decided to text Grace, my doula. Grace thought it was likely my water as the liquid didn't smell like pee.

I called my midwifery office and learned that Laura was the midwife on call that weekend. Laura told me that it sounded like my mucous plug had come out and my water had indeed broken, but to come in mid-day for her to check. I hadn't been feeling any sensations. I decided to take a long, hot shower. We then called my parents and gave them a heads up that they should start the four hour drive to our house now since I was in early labor. We dropped the girls off at our friends' house while we went to see the midwives.

It had been about four hours since my water had broken at 8:00am. I still wasn't feeling any sensations aside from mild cramping. I wasn't even timing the cramping as it was so sporadic and mild. Although I am not a donut person, my husband and I have a tradition of going to Dunkin Donuts when I am in early labor. We had done it with both of our older girls, so we had to do it with Indie too! I asked my husband to get me an iced coffee -- fully caffeinated as I was expecting a long day and evening ahead of us!

We arrived at the birthing center at noon and Laura immediately took me into an exam room and confirmed that my water had broken. The midwives don't check for dilation this early on in labor as it can create unnecessary anxiety for mom to find out she isn't even dilated. Plus, Laura could see based on my appearance that I really wasn't very far along at this point. But she did say, "We'll be meeting this baby later tonight." That got me excited. I knew today or tomorrow would be the day we met our third daughter!

Because nothing was progressing, Laura sent us home and suggested we should do things to help naturally start labor. She suggested lots of walking and nipple stimulation. If I didn't go into active labor by 8:00am on Monday, I'd have to go the hospital for an induction. Given how much I wanted to have an unmedicated birth in the birthing center, I decided I'd do everything I could possibly do to avoid an induction.

As soon as we got home, we went for a walk around the lake in our community. My contractions weren't getting any stronger and in fact were nearly non-existent. I held out hope that tonight would be the night. While walking, I took in the sounds of nature around me. The birds chirping and the glorious fall day warmed my soul.

My parents arrived around 3:00pm. During this time my mom and I went for another walk around the lake. We saw some people while walking and I decided not to mention to anyone that I was in early labor, despite everyone asking me how I was feeling. Most knew that my due date was Halloween. There was something inside me that was afraid to mention I was in early labor. I wanted to keep her and I safe from feeling the pressure and anticipation of giving birth.

As the afternoon progressed, I started to feel like my contractions were increasing, but I was still easily able to go about my daily business. I called Laura to give her an update and she encouraged me to sleep and call her back when my contractions were five minutes apart and lasting for one minute each.

I had arranged for my parents to take the girls Trick or Treating with some friends so my husband and I could stay home and relax. We even put a bucket of candy outside so we didn't have to socialize with anyone. I felt myself starting to retreat. I just wanted to curl up on the couch and watch something happy on TV. We put on HGTV while the kids were out Trick or Treating.

The girls and my parents returned home around 7:30pm and it became very chaotic in our house. It was loud and the girls were energized to show us all the candy they had collected. I felt my body and mind shifting for labor. I just wanted to crawl into bed, rest quietly, and relax my body and mind. Prior to going to bed, I told both girls that it was unlikely they'd see me in the morning because I'd probably be having their sister tonight. I kissed both girls and told them I loved them. I sensed that my 9-year-old was nervous, so I reassured her that Mommy and Indie would be in safe hands and we'd be home soon with her baby sister!

I woke up around 11:00pm to the strongest sensations yet. I started to time them, but they were not even close to having a pattern, so I stopped. I was too excited and anxious to go back to sleep. I laid in bed until 12:30am and it was during this time that I felt my sensations began to take on a consistent pattern. Indie was really starting to speak to me! I woke my husband up and told him I thought it was time to go even though my contractions were more like 45 seconds long as opposed to 1 minute. Instinctively I knew it was time to get to the birthing center.

My husband took care of calling both Laura and Grace to let them know what was going on. Laura told us to come in at 2:00am. I kissed both girls in bed before we left. My 9-year-old happened to be awake and was feeling anxious. I told her that her sister was on her way, and we'd be home sometime tomorrow. (The birthing center policy is to discharge mom and baby around 4-6 hours after birth). I would later learn that she laid in bed for the next couple of hours crying and woke my mom up at 4:00am to talk to her. It turns out they were awake together at 4:32 when Indie was born!

We arrived at the birthing center at 2:00 on the dot. Grace pulled in at the same time we did. I gave her a hug. A nurse greeted us at the front door and guided me to an exam room so Laura could check me. When Laura checked me, I was 5 centimeters dilated and she told me we'd be staying and meeting our baby in the coming hours. There were two other families there that night and I got the last available room – phew!

Once we got settled into the room, Laura and the nurse gave us some time alone for me to labor with the support of Grace and my husband. My sensations started to pick up in intensity, so Grace showed my husband the "hip squeeze," where he basically applied a lot of pressure outside my hips and pushed in. This felt really good as it somewhat relieved the strong sensations I was starting to feel in my low back.

I sat on the toilet for a bit because I remembered it feeling so good with my second daughter's homebirth, but this time around it didn't feel good AT ALL. I decided I wanted to walk around the birthing center, so we went out into the main area. I think we even walked through the kitchen, which is when I remember Laura telling us that because of Covid, we had to stay in our room. It was at that point that I vomited. I recall hearing Laura say, "She's transitioning," and that's when I knew we'd be meeting Indie soon!

We took the few short steps back into our room and that's when I remember losing my senses. I really went inward at this point. I just wanted to be leaning over the bed where I found the most relief. My husband and Grace continued to squeeze my hips through each sensation. There would come a point during each one where I would yell stop. I just kept looking forward to the break between the sensations where I could catch my breath and restore my focus. I had begun making extremely primal sounds. They sounded really intense to me. These sounds brought me relief and got me out of my head. It was purely instinctual. It is incredible what the female body is capable of under such intense circumstances like giving birth. I am reminded that we are animals at our core.

Grace was feeding me ice chips in between the contractions, and I found these to be both refreshing in my mouth but also an opportunity to return to the human world of eating something from a spoon. I think eating the ice chips off a spoon also served as a reminder that I was still alive during the most intense sensations my body had ever felt. Each time I had an ice chip it reminded me I had made it through a sensation and that was incredibly motivating for me.

I remember Laura coming in and saying she'd be checking my dilation in between the next contraction and I begged her not to. I was feeling so much sensation in my rectum that even the thought of her putting her fingers into my vagina was quite frankly, terrifying. I was also scared she might report back that I had not progressed in terms of dilation. I allowed her to check me though, and she said I was 9 centimeters dilated! I was so relieved to hear this.

Then I started to no longer get any relief between sensations. It was like one long sensation. I told Laura I felt the urge to push and she encouraged me to let my body ride and go with that feeling. Laura was massaging my calves at this point and it felt so good. Again, I think feeling hands on my calves, even just a gentle massage, brought me back earthside for a few seconds here and there because so much of me during this time was in a totally different realm. I continued with my primal sounds. They were LOUD. I remember Laura telling me to go low and deep, so that's what I did. She also had me sink my bum to my heels, so gravity could help push Indie out.

When I felt a burning sensation, I knew that was the ring of fire. Laura told me she could see her head. It felt like my husband had been quiet for a while and it was now that I said to him, "Please just remind me you're here. I just want to know you're here with me." Once I got that confirmation from him, I pushed. I pushed about three times and then I felt Indie squeeze through and out of my vagina. It's the most incredible feeling in the entire world, feeling your child exit your body.

I immediately flipped over and onto my back so I could see our beautiful baby girl. Indie was placed on my chest, and we laid skin to skin for a long time while Laura and the nurse monitored both of our vitals. She'd soon nuzzle her way up to one of my breasts and practice nursing. My husband was able to cut her chord after a several minute chord clamping delay. I then delivered the placenta and Laura determined I needed 1 stitch.

The three of us lay in the birthing center bed and bonded for the next few hours. We worked on her latch, which turned out to be harder than it was with my two older girls, but we managed to get her on for some colostrum. I even dozed off to sleep. The nurses checked our vitals often but were able to do so in a way that didn't interrupt our sleep or family bonding time. It was a quiet and magical time.

We called my parents and older daughters at 7:30am to speak with them on the phone. I was so relieved to share the news with the girls and my parents as I had been feeling quite a bit of anxiety in the weeks leading up to Indie's birth. All I wanted was to know that our baby was healthy, and she was!

We decided to send the girls to school that day so we could have several hours alone with Indie before she met her two older sisters. The three of us were discharged 4 hours after Indie was born. We went home, had coffee, and crawled into bed.

Indie met her big sisters later that afternoon. I'll never forget the HUGE smiles on their faces as they ran into the house to meet and snuggle with their baby sister! I cried, absolutely delighted to be in the arms of each of my children.

November 4, 2021

Abby and Rylan

In December 2020, a few days before Christmas, I woke Scott up and waved a pregnancy test in his face telling him to wake up and that I was pregnant. We were so excited! We enjoyed the holidays with family, without telling them. A few days later, I started bleeding. I had a gut feeling, and I knew what was happening. I spent days crying and crying and asking God why. I had experienced my first miscarriage, and I was heartbroken. We decided to keep trying and we cleaned up our lifestyle so much. My family and friends thought we were crazy.

Two months later, on March 1, I got my positive pregnancy test. On that same day, we went straight to the birthing center to confirm with a blood test and check my progesterone. It was confirmed, and we were rushed with so many emotions: happiness, anxiety, and worry. The first trimester in pregnancy is scary, especially after a loss.

I already knew I wanted Morgan to be my doula. This was planned even in the early weeks of the first baby we lost. She was with me through the loss and into this pregnancy. We spoke about my birth plans and I had decided to use a Birth Center. Morgan wanted to support whatever I wanted for my birth and was ready to help me have the most beautiful water birth ever!

I started doing a lot of research on things I wanted for my birth plan. I followed a lot of moms on Instagram and watched and read their testimonials about their experiences. I saw so many videos and pictures of the most beautiful home births. When I was 20 weeks, I decided that I needed to have this baby at home. It's really hard to explain, but I just had a moment of, "I need to do this and I trust my body so much." I talked it over with Scott, and he said what I knew he was going to say. It was my body, and he fully trusted the decision I wanted to make to birth our child. So, I started searching for a midwife. I called a few different women, asked a lot of questions, and ultimately decided on a woman who I instantly connected with. I look back now and could never imagine having someone different.

I continued prenatal care with my midwife and saw her once a month, and more often closer to my due date. Our appointments were an hour or more each visit, and we were able to discuss so many things. Every test, swab, and decision was left completely up to me. This was the biggest difference in care. I was able to make my own decisions for my baby and my body. Whether it be intuition based, or evidence based, it was all left for me to decide.

As we got closer to my due date, we started to explain to Mason about the birthing process. We wanted him to be home for the birth. If he wanted to be in the room, that was something we would leave entirely up to him. Him being home was important to us for bonding. We taught him words like "uterus" and "amniotic fluid." We told him I would be in pain, and probably making weird noises. Whether or not he'll ever remember this, that's okay. I just wanted him to know that birth was a normal part of life, and how beautiful it really is. His interest level was about one on a scale of one to ten.

Morgan and I had plans to make the most beautiful birthing space in my room. We planned on putting beautiful lights in the pool, setting up candles, and stringing my affirmation cards around the room. I dreamed of this beautiful birthing spot for months and months. I was going to have my hair in the cutest braids. Kristen, my photographer, was going to come and capture it all on camera. I had my playlist all ready. I couldn't wait for the day. I was craving the experience.

The Monday after Halloween, around 4:00pm, I was lying in my bed watching TV when I felt the smallest gush in my underwear. I got up because I knew it couldn't have been urine, but it also wasn't enough to be my water breaking. I had seen movies and TV shows and listened to other women talk about this "huge waterfall" when their water broke. I just knew it couldn't have been my water. I texted my midwife, and she told me to use a Q-TIP that I had in my birth kit to test for amniotic fluid. I swabbed it and sent her a picture, and she responded, "Well, your water just broke." My immediate response was "That wasn't very movie-like."

My midwife called me and told me to eat a nice nourishing meal with tons of protein and to get some good rest. I texted Scott and told him that my water had broken. He came home from work, and we set up everything we needed. We got the pool set up and Scott and my mom braided my hair. We moved the table with all the things my midwife needed, and we also moved the bed. We then went to sleep thinking we were going to have a baby that night.

I woke up the next morning with no change, except I was losing a lot more fluid. It was filling pads and dripping EVERYWHERE, but still no contractions. I knew that my water could be broken for 72 hours before a small risk of infection happened, so I continued to let my body ride it out. Honestly, at this point, I was willing to go over 72 hours because I knew the baby would come when they were ready. My midwife told me about a midwives' brew that I could drink to try and naturally get things going. I wasn't ready to do anything to my body to bring on labor and the brew was going to be my last resort. Tuesday came and went with no contractions. I woke up Wednesday morning with still no contractions and no change. I had never had any cervical checks and had zero idea how dilated I was or what my cervix was like. I was just going to trust my body.

That Wednesday morning, I woke up with still no contractions, just still losing a lot of fluid. I went to see Julie in the afternoon. Julie is the pelvic floor specialist that I see that specializes in body work. I went to see her to try and open up some space for the baby to come out. We also used magnets on some pressure points. She said that a lot of women start contracting while they are there at the center, so I kept thinking that it would be the day. But again, nothing happened. We went home and continued to go about our day, wondering if every Braxton Hicks contraction was the start of labor. It was not.

Thursday morning, I woke up with still no contractions. I met my midwife to check the baby's heartbeat and get some herbs. We discussed the midwives brew again. At 4:00pm that day, it would be 72 hours since my water had broken. On the ride home from the midwife's house, Scott and I discussed the brew recipe she gave me. We weighed out our options and risk factors, and I decided I would drink it. My personal comfort level of risk and mental health was dwindling, and I knew I would need a strong mind for labor.

Scott took the dog to the groomer, went to the store, and then mixed up the drink for me. This was about 1:30. The midwives brew typically brings on labor in 4-6 hours if your body is ready. I drank the drink and sat on my exercise ball. I also used my pump a little bit. Scott left to pick the dog back up and get Mason from the bus stop. I texted him at about 2:00pm and told him that I thought I had maybe felt some contractions, but I wasn't sure if these were "baby producing contractions." I had never felt them with Mason because I had an epidural with him.

My midwife texted me around 3:00 and said to try and take a nap if I was able. I got in my bed, and it was almost immediately that I started having labor contractions. I started to time them and they were very inconsistent. Some were two minutes apart, some were one, and some were thirteen. I was texting with Morgan and told her I would let her know when I was ready for her to come. I remembered my midwife said to call her when they were "5-1-1." Five minutes apart, lasting one minute, for one hour.

The contractions had only been going on for about 20 minutes, and the times were so sporadic. The contractions eventually started to get worse in the bed, so I asked Scott to fill up the bathtub so I could sit in the hot water and work through my contractions. I kept saying, "I just need to poop! I just really need to poop." I got into the bathtub and had him play my playlist, and I sat for a bit. It was time for Scott to tell Morgan and Kristen (the photographer) to come over.

I was sitting on my back in the tub, and Scott kept saying, "Let's flip you over, and get you off your back," and I kept saying, "No!" I finally flipped over to my hands and knees because he reminded me that I made it clear I didn't want to birth on my back. He started to attempt to fill up the birthing pool so we could make the beautiful space I wanted. I remember my sister had just walked in and said hello. She had come to be with Mason, who was at the neighbor's house.

The contractions started getting super intense, so I yelled to Scott to turn the music off. With every contraction, I kept screaming, "I EITHER HAVE TO POOP OR THIS BABY IS COMING!" Scott was on the phone with my midwife, and she told him that if I didn't feel the urge to push, try not to. I vividly remember screaming, "YOU TELL HER THAT I HAVE TO PUSH, AND SHE CAN'T KEEP SAYING THAT." But she didn't know how close I was and was trying to help me prevent tearing. She was on the phone watching me work through contractions. Morgan finally arrived, and at this point I was on my hands and knees pushing. She came in and attempted to light some candles and try and set the pool up, but it was too late. She sat beside the tub with me and poured some warm water on my back. I kept saying, "Y'all this baby is coming." Scott kept saying that he didn't think it was time yet.

With one contraction, I looked at Morgan and I screamed, "He's coming!" She told me to reach down to see if I could feel his head, and sure enough I could. That's when I knew I was about to have this baby right now in the bathtub. I SCREAMED for Scott to get in there because he was still trying to fill the birthing pool. By this time, my baby was halfway out. My husband and my sister came into the bathroom, and I told them he was coming. Morgan told them to get ready to catch him. Scott got down behind me, my sister grabbed a towel, and out he came with the last push.

He was welcomed into this world by his dad and his aunt, Anna-Grace. His cord was so long it was wrapped around his leg! Morgan unwrapped the cord, and we maneuvered my body so I could get back on my back. Then they handed me my sweet little boy. He wasn't crying at all. He was SO calm! I kept asking if he was okay, and I realized that he was perfect. My midwife kept an eye on me through the phone, checking our color. I immediately latched him onto my breast, and we sat in the tub for a while. I was waiting for my placenta to come out, but it was stubborn. I told my sister to run and get Mason, so he could see that his brother was just born. He walked into a bathtub full of blood, and a baby still attached to his mom. His response was, "Okay I'm going back to play."

My midwife finally walked in, took a look at us, and said everything looked perfect. I decided to get up with the baby still attached to me, so that I could try and deliver the placenta while comfy in my bed. Kristen had just gotten there in time to capture the delivery of the placenta. The pain of trying to deliver the placenta was 100 times worse than labor. I kept him breastfeeding, hoping the placenta would release. I started bleeding more than normal. I made it very clear that if I was to bleed, I wanted herbs to stop the bleeding. She told me I was bleeding pretty heavily and gave me some tinctures. I kept asking if I was okay. She reassured me I was fine, but she was keeping an eye on the bleeding. It had been well over an hour, and my placenta was not coming out. I was starting to bleed even more. She told me I had lost a liter of blood, and if I kept bleeding. I was going to need something to stop the bleeding. I kept telling her that I didn't want anything.

The bleeding had gotten worse with every push for the placenta. She looked at me and said, "Do you trust me? You need something to stop the bleeding." I vividly remember looking at Morgan for some reassurance, and she nodded her head up and down, and I told my midwife okay. She wanted to prevent a transfer, or any postpartum complications. I obviously wasn't too happy, but I had learned to trust her this whole journey enough to tell me I needed something to keep me safe. My placenta finally came out, about an hour and a half or more later.

Scott finally cut the cord and I sat in bed while Scott and my midwife fed me a medium rare steak and a baked potato from Outback. After everyone left, we slowly drifted off to sleep in our own bed with our newborn and our 8 year old on a pallet at the foot of the bed, watching a movie. No bright lights, no doctors coming in and out, no pokes, and no goop. Just mom, dad, and our new baby asleep in the very place he was made!

Although I didn't get my beautiful room set up with my pool and lights, it was the most perfect home birth. The feeling I felt right when he came out of my body is indescribable. I felt a high I had never felt before. I felt so proud of my body and proud of Scott for trusting me to have this experience. Pregnancy made me so aware of my body, and I will forever be thankful for how I learned to use my voice. I will forever be grateful for the things I learned about birth and babies.

Whether you want to birth in a hospital, a birthing center, your home, a train or a plane, I want you to know that your body was made to birth your sweet baby. Always remember that you are capable and strong, and always fight for what you know you can do

November 6, 2021

Amber and Beau

I woke up around 8:00am to the faint sound of giggles and morning clatter. My husband had been getting up with the kids every morning for months, letting me sleep in. I had light contractions, inconsistently spaced and 10 minutes apart. As I laid in bed I decided to meditate. I had never meditated before in my life, but I had a birthing app with some preloaded ones, so I gave it a try. Forty minutes passed in what felt like only five, and at that point I started to think, "Today just might be the day."

I went out to join Brandon and the kids and let him know how I was feeling. We went about our morning as normal. I was fluttering around the house picking up. Putting clean sheets on the bed, wiping down the kitchen, making sure the fridge was stocked with the essentials for Carson and Juliette. I was feeling a bit of last minute nesting. By 10:00 I let my mom and Brandon's mom know what was going on. Contractions were still nearly 10 minutes apart. It was difficult to gauge when to tell out of town family to head on over. The contractions could mean a baby in five hours or five days. By 11:00

the contractions were 2-3 minutes apart, still low intensity, but I knew it was happening. We called the birth team. My incredible midwives, Nancy and Isabelle, along with our phenomenal photographer, Carey, started to head over.

Nancy arrived first with all her supplies in tow. It was such a warm feeling to know that she trusted me and my body, while at the same time had everything we could need if there were to be an emergency. Brandon was on his way home with turkey subs and strawberries. It seemed silly to send him on an errand at such a time, but a solid lunch was needed and strawberries are the go to snack for our kids. We couldn't be without those on such a day!

Nancy, Isabelle, and Carey got our bedroom and bathroom all set up. The had supplies organized, towels placed all cute, and bedding turned down. At this point everything was ready to go and we just got to hang out and chat while my contractions get closer together. We were all in the kitchen and Isabelle asked if I'd like her to fill the tub. I wasn't sure it was really that time yet. Contractions were still pretty mild, but they were only a minute or so apart. I'm thankful she suggested it when she did. By the time the tub was full I was ready to get in.

I started off leaning back. Juliette stayed right with me, stroking my arm, hugging me. She said, "Hi," to each person with her sweet little grin countless times. Carson was in and out of the bathroom, pleasantly calm and supportive when he was near me. Brandon was attentively watching and ready for anything I might need, but he never hovered or crowded me. He knows me well. After some time, I really couldn't tell you how long, the intensity picked up. I moved into a crouched squat position which helped. It still felt very intense, but I no longer had to fight against gravity. I think my mom arrived around this time. I remember hearing the kids laugh and play in the background. It was music to my ears and warmth to my soul.

At this point I finally started to push. I had been waiting and trying to just breathe through each contraction. I wanted to let my body move Beau down without me straining too early on. But now, it was time. I had Brandon come close to hold my hand. The other hand was on the bottom of the tub for support. I would get Beau so close and then he would retreat. The thoughts of, "I can't do this" tried to break through, but I would override them with, "Your body is made for this." I was feeling empowered and defeated at the same time.

I started wondering, "Why haven't I gotten this baby out yet? I'm prepared! I've prepared my mind, I've prepared my body. What's the deal?" Then I got my answer. Nancy was able to see that he was still in the sac. Through all this laboring my water never broke. I was working down my baby who was still inside this balloon. This gave me some relief because I felt validated that yes this was hard, and dang it hurts, and here's the reason why. Then the sac broke, but his hands were up by his face. He'd had the freedom to move around instead of his arms being pinned at his sides. I heard Nancy excitedly say, "He just grabbed my finger!" It makes me smile to think back on Beau wrapping his tiny fist around her finger before being born. My next push brought Beau earth-side.

The immediate sense of relief, gratitude, and zero pain is pretty incredible. That natural birth high you hear about is true. I remember holding him on my chest and thinking how big he was! And how much gorgeous vernix was all over him. And his hair! He was here. Finally here.

Nancy had me get out of the water within a few minutes. I had some bleeding and she wanted to be able to see better and make sure it wasn't too much, which was difficult to do in water. When I stood to get out, she held Beau to my chest to keep him on me, the importance of skin to skin honored and protected. We moved to my bed and everything was fine. Beau nursed for the first time. Carson cut the cord. Juliette snuggled in close. Brandon was near, loving and supportive.

My mom went to grab dinner. Nancy insisted on me eating a full meal and I'm glad she did. I was exhausted and needed fuel. I shared a bowl of spaghetti with my daughter, in my bed, while my newborn baby got his exam done. There were no tears, no screaming, no measurements done moments after birth, no cold plastic box. He was calm, warm, nursed, and didn't mind being weighed and measured. During his exam she noticed he had lip, tongue, and cheek ties. She gave me contact information for the best tie revision doctor in the valley and we got them fixed when he was two days old. His latch immediately improved. He nursed like a champ!

Nancy and Isabelle stayed and got us all settled, cleaned up the bathroom, and soaked towels in hydrogen peroxide to get the blood out. By the time they left it was bedtime for Carson and Jules and my mom and mother-in-law got them off to bed. Brandon and I got to just stare at our third miracle and reminisce on the day.

I don't think I slept more than an hour that night. Not because of a crying baby, I just couldn't stop staring at him! I had this energy even though I knew I should be exhausted. I liked the feeling of being the only one awake in the house. Just me, able to soak in my baby all to myself.

This experience was like nothing else. I loved having my children present. My son was able to witness the strength of women and see first-hand a physiological birth. My daughter was able to see what she will be capable of someday and to trust her intuition.

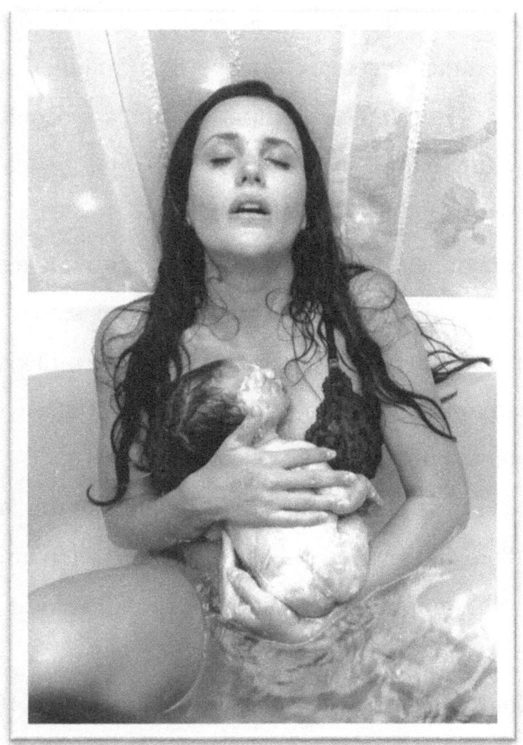

Photo by Carey Lauren
Carey Lauren Photos & Film

November 9, 2021

Esther and Lily: A Birth in Texas

I started having contractions Monday night from 11:00pm until 4:00am. When they were 5 minutes apart, I called my wonderful doula and she headed to our home from an hour away. When she arrived at 5:00am, my contractions spaced out to 8-10 minutes apart, then 20 minutes, then 30-50 minutes. Around 1:30pm we decided she would leave for a little while so we could nap, get rested, and see if contractions would come back without her there.

Almost immediately they started coming closer again. I called my doula back and while on the phone with her I started averaging 4 minutes apart and they were intense. I called the midwives, and they told us to head to the birth center. Forty minutes later we arrived and then time became blurry.

I had a cervical check and was 4 centimeters dilated and 90% effaced. I walked and swayed outside while doing hip circles. I passed an egg sized clot after they checked me. At 6:20 I said I needed to go back inside.

I was checked again and was 5.5 centimeters and 100% effaced. I passed another egg sized clot, so we did a stress test. It was horrible having to sit for the stress test while my contractions were so close together. The stress test said everything was good and they determined the clots were from how fast my cervix was changing. I got admitted and I took a long warm shower and did hip circles and some squats. I started feeling pressure and the urge to push with contractions. I felt my water bulging between my hips.

After the shower I got out and my midwife asked to check me on the bed, but I needed to squat. She saw me trying to push, so my midwife squatted down with me and felt that baby was at station 0, fully effaced and I was 8 centimeters dilated. It was time to get in the birth tub.

I got in on hands and knees and would move to squatting with my knees closed. My midwife suggested I roll over and float because I was trying to push too much between contractions. I floated and would move back to my knees during contractions. I would breathe with an open jaw, relax my shoulders, and lock eyes with my sweet husband, my mom, my doula, and my midwife. I made horse noises to help release tension.

One time when I was belly up and semi-floating in the water, my water bag began to bulge and then burst! My baby dropped even further and started to crown. I lost it for a moment, but they helped keep me grounded. My fast contractions and pushing was stressing the baby a little bit. Because of the stress, my midwife said we needed to get out of tub and go sideways on the bed. She suggested a position that would help keep baby's heart rate stable.

At 10:16pm I gave birth to my little one and one of my awesome midwives caught her! She came out with a hand first, then her head facing my back. She was like a Supergirl! We left her attached and about 30 minutes later we cut the cord. I accepted a Pitocin injection for bleeding and to help my placenta come out. It came out and they inspected it. It was fully intact.

My birth team got consent for everything. They explained each procedure. They cared about my goal to avoid trauma for baby and me while doing everything in their power to help me labor safely and birth my baby safely. I felt like I had been to war and I was a warrior. It was amazing. And squishy, cuddly, sweet baby Lily is my prize.

November 10, 2021

Sarah and Jacob: A Birth in Vermont

I went to my 39 week prenatal appointment on Tuesday, November 9th. It was at the appointment that I discovered I was presenting with high blood pressure. My OB decided it would be best for me to head to Labor and Delivery for monitoring and told me there was a high chance I would need to be induced. I continued to present high blood pressure readings, which had my team worried I had preeclampsia. After blood and urine were sampled, it was determined I did not have preeclampsia, but was diagnosed with gestational hypertension. My OB wanted me to be induced to prevent preeclampsia. I called Mark and told him to grab our bags and head to the hospital to meet me. I was devastated I needed to be induced and thought it would lead to outcomes I had not hoped for my birth.

A foley catheter and misoprostol were placed around 8:30pm to dilate and ripen my cervix. I was given a second dose of misoprostol at 11:30pm and a third dose at 2:30am. The foley came out around 5:30am when I was dilated to 4 centimeters. I was having frequent contractions, but they were not strong, and I did not feel them. I was started on Pitocin around 7:45am and was dilated to 5 centimeters around 8:30am. At this time my OB wanted to break my waters, which I consented to.

I spent a lot of time in early labor on the birth ball. Then I moved to standing with my head tucked into Mark's chest squeezing his biceps and rocking rhythmically when contractions picked up. I asked my nurse to call the volunteer doula in at this point. Emma was such an amazing asset to have at my birth.

After some time, I decided to labor in the tub. It provided so much relief. I squeezed two combs in my hands or squeezed Mark's hand while in the peak of my contractions. I tapped my right foot really fast to distract myself from the intensity. Mark had to remind me to breathe deeply and slowly to stay grounded and present in the moment. I labored in the tub for about 20 minutes before I could feel the baby coming and the need to push.

I had to use short quick breaths to avoid pushing. I had to get out of the tub and labor through three contractions before I made it to the bed. This was NOT easy! I was dilated to 10 centimeters at 11:29am and was told hair could be seen and it was time to push! I pushed for 30 minutes and my baby was born at 11:59am. Mark announced that we had a baby boy! Jacob Thomas St. Pierre was 8.1 pounds, 21.5 inches long and absolutely perfect.

After being disappointed that I needed to be induced, I was pleasantly surprised that almost all of my labor wishes were still able to be followed and that I was able to give birth without any pain management! I got the quick labor and vaginal delivery that I desired. It was an amazing experience and I am so thankful to have had a happy birth and healthy baby.

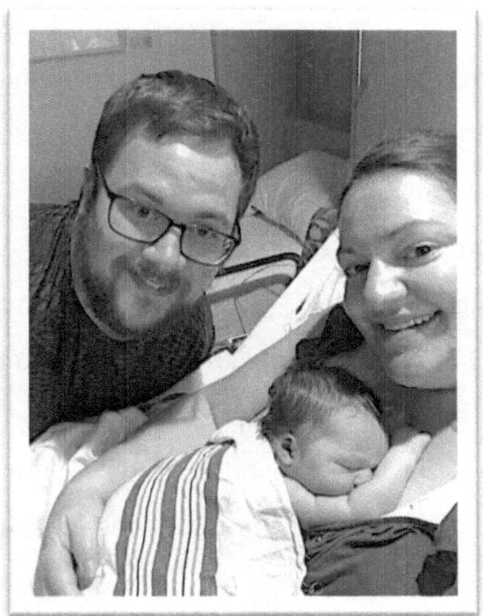

Sarah and Quinn: A Birth in Vermont

When I was pregnant with my third baby, I fell into the trap of comparing her birth date to my previous pregnancies. My first baby came three days "late", my second baby came three days "early", and I thought for sure that this baby would come even earlier. She was feeling so heavy and large, and I had been having painful Braxton Hicks since about 25 weeks. I had invited my sister, Katie, to come up from New York City and witness the birth of her niece and be our birth photographer. She arrived when I was 39 weeks pregnant and planned to stay for a week. I thought surely I would have this baby sometime during the 39th week of pregnancy...

But my baby was very comfortable and had no interest in being born. Katie postponed her flight home three different times, but had to get back to work soon. I had prodromal labor every night, but by 2:00am the contractions would stop, and I would go to sleep. Then every morning I would wake up feeling frustrated that labor hadn't started. Katie moved her flight one last time and had to fly home on the tenth. So, on Tuesday the 9th, I decided to drink some castor oil and see if I could get the prodromal labor to turn into actual labor.

My midwife was comfortable with me taking castor oil and said she would come over to check in with me when she was done her prenatal visits that Tuesday evening. After choking down some castor oil mixed in with scrambled eggs and cheese, my husband, Kyle, Katie, and I watched some TV and anxiously waited to see if anything would happen. I sat on an exercise ball and did hip circles while we watched. My midwife, Jen, arrived around 7:30pm and brought her assistant, Sienna, with her. When nothing seemed to be happening, Jen suggested we try to get some sleep. She and Sienna slept on the couches in the living room, and we all headed to bed.

Kyle and I got to our room, and I expressed my frustration that nothing seemed to be happening. I was feeling really defeated and sad that our baby was taking so long. I tried my best to get some rest, but soon after I laid down the castor oil started working in the way it is intended to – and I spent the next hour making trips back and forth to the bathroom to poop. Once I stopped using the bathroom around 11:00, I was ready to try and sleep. But as soon as I was tired enough and had given up on labor starting, the contractions started. It felt just like the prodromal labor I had been having for weeks, but by 2:00am the contractions continued instead of stopping. I was so excited that I went out to tell Jen that I thought labor might be happening!

I went back to bed and tried to rest while Kyle snored next to me. I knew he needed rest, and the contractions were very mild. I really enjoyed laying in the dark and feeling my baby move and just easily breathing through each contraction as it came. I was so excited to meet the little person that was growing inside.

Around 5:00am the contractions became painful enough that I wanted to get out of bed. I woke up Kyle and we went out to the living room where we could have more space to move around. Jen and Sienna went into our older kids' rooms to continue trying to rest and give us some space. Our older two kids were staying with my parents while we prepared for labor. I knew from my previous labors that I tend to swear a lot and don't like distractions. I knew I would be happier laboring without them around.

We woke up Katie and she joined us. I was enjoying leaning over our kitchen island during the contractions. Kyle put air in the birth pool so it would be ready when I wanted it filled. We were all excited, but labor didn't seem to be progressing very quickly. I laid down on the couch around 7:00am because I hadn't gotten any sleep and was feeling so sleepy. When I laid down it was as if labor stopped. I held Kyle's hand and fell asleep. I woke up at 8:30 and Jen asked how I was doing. I was confused because the contractions had been so steady and then seemed to completely stop. She asked if I wanted a cervical check and I said yes. I was 5-6 centimeters dilated and was reassured that I would probably meet my baby that day.

Once I was up, the contractions came back. I never timed them or timed how far apart they were. I just listened to my body and focused on opening. I ate some breakfast and continued to lean over the kitchen counter for contractions. Kyle would rub my back and squeeze my hips. He was such an amazing support for me. In between contractions we would all talk and laugh and enjoy each other's company. It was such a fun morning.

During each contraction I would visualize my cervix opening and picture my uterus squeezing my baby down. This kind of visualization had been so helpful to me during my last birth, and it was helpful again this time. I found the contractions were never too hard to get through when I kept my focus on what was physically happening inside my body. Remembering that the contractions were just my body doing the work of labor for me was really helpful.

Around 10:00am, Kyle, Katie, and I went to walk outside. We live on a quiet dirt road with views of the mountains, and it was surprisingly warm in Vermont for November. We didn't walk very fast or very far, but the sunshine felt so nice. When I would feel a contraction coming, Kyle would bend at the waist and allow me to lean onto him for support. I knew labor was progressing now, and after a short walk I wanted to go back inside. I was ready to get into water and Jen said we could start to fill the pool if I wanted.

Sienna helped Kyle and Katie fill the pool. I leaned over the counter while I waited for the relief of the warm water. I snacked on crackers and string cheese and made sure to be drinking water in between contractions. Getting in the water felt amazing. I remember taking the hose and letting the water flow over my belly. Kyle sat outside the pool holding my hands, rubbing my shoulders, and pushing on my lower back. I loved the water and kept changing positions as I felt myself opening. I would lean over the edge of the pool for a few contractions, then I would sit back and try to relax for the next few. I honestly don't know how long I was in the pool for. Time got very blurry.

I started to feel the pressure that I knew meant my baby was coming soon. It was so intense, and I knew I could push through the pressure, but the thought of pushing seemed too painful. I reached a finger down and I could feel my bag of water and my baby's head right inside. She was so close, but I wasn't ready to push. I moaned and swore through the contractions and took deep slow breaths. During the moments between contractions, my baby would move and wiggle. It was so special to feel her moving and know that she was working with me to be born. We were in this together. I trusted her to help me when it was the right time.

The pressure got very intense, but the water in the pool was just cold enough that I didn't want to be in it anymore. I knew it was almost time for her to be born and I went to go labor on the toilet. We have a small bathroom that our kids use, and it felt safe and comfortable to be in that space. Jen reassured me that she has seen a lot of babies born in bathrooms. She waited in the hallway while Kyle and I went into the bathroom. Kyle sat on the edge of the tub and held my hand and rubbed my thigh while I had a couple of contractions on the toilet. After two contractions there, I knew my baby was coming.

"I feel the pushing urge," I said.

"That's great," said Jen, coming into the room, "You're doing great."

I knelt down next to the toilet with one knee down and one knee up in a half squat. Kyle sat behind me on the edge of the tub, holding me and telling me how amazing I was doing. My body completely took over at this point. I reached a hand down and felt my baby's head starting to be born. I wasn't pushing - if anything I was trying to hold her back. I whispered to my baby, "slow down," as she started to crown. I had allowed my body the space and time to do the work for me, and my body pushed entirely on its own. My water broke in a splash right before her head was born. Her body followed seconds later in the same contraction. She was born with her hands next to her face.

Jen helped catch her as she came flying out and immediately she was on my chest. It happened so quickly, and I was amazed at what my body just did. Feeling the fetal ejection reflex was like an out of body experience. She came out pink and screaming. I held her to me and talked to her. Kyle and I admired the perfect little girl we had created. We named her Quinn Katherine.

My placenta detached and was birthed a few minutes after Quinn was born. I had a bit more bleeding than normal, and agreed to have a shot of Pitocin. Quinn laid in my arms while Jen checked for any tearing. I did not need any stitches. I gave Quinn and her placenta to Kyle to hold, and he went to lay skin-to-skin with her in our bed. I got cleaned up and then went to bed to join them. Kyle and I laid with Quinn and she nursed for the first time. Jen and Sienna emptied the pool and cleaned up in the living room while giving us time together to meet our baby. It was so comfortable to be snuggled in our bed.

After about an hour, Jen came in and asked if we were ready for the newborn exam. I stayed tucked into bed and Jen laid Quinn next to me to measure her and take her weight. She was exactly 9 pounds. My biggest baby yet. Kyle cut the umbilical cord and we put Quinn's placenta in the freezer to make prints with later. Katie had postponed her flight one last time while I was in labor, but had to leave soon to catch her flight home. We said goodbye to Jen and Sienna, and then said goodbye to Katie. I stayed tucked in bed for the next few hours cuddling and nursing my new baby. Kyle brought me food and more water. That first night we slept in our own bed with Quinn right beside us. She has filled our lives with so much happiness and joy ever since.

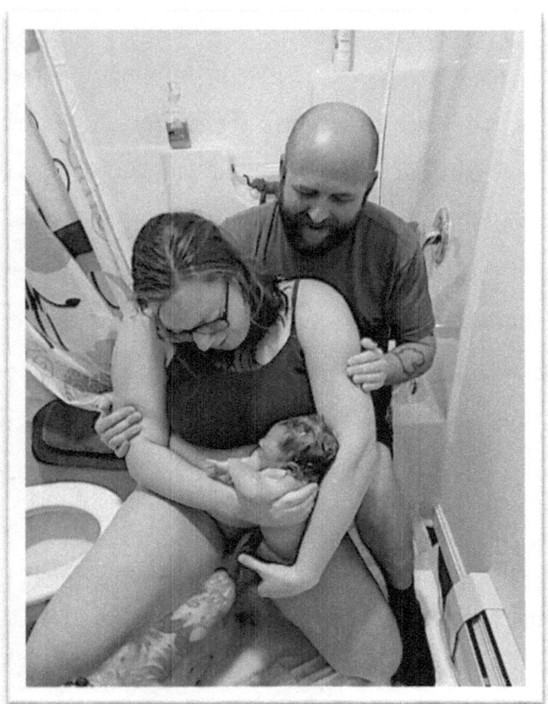

November 12, 2021

Megan and Crosby

November 11, 2021, I felt my first contraction ever. I was pregnant with my third child and was extremely excited and eager to experience my first vaginal birth. My older children were both delivered via C-Section because my doctors at the time were not comfortable with delivering a breech or VBAC baby. For my third and last child I craved redemption through a non-medicated home birth.

I was 6 days past my due date. Part of me doubted that my body could actually go into labor because I had never reached that point in pregnancy before. I patiently waited. My homebirth team assured me that when my mind and body felt it was safe and ready, the process would begin. It was a Thursday and my husband, Nick's, first day off in seven days. He was home, I felt safe, I felt strong, and I was ready. I had mild but true contractions all day. Once our children were asleep, the contractions were consistently 9 minutes apart and getting stronger. I got in a warm bath with Nick sitting next to the tub holding my hand. We smiled at each other and were so excited with anticipation for what this new experience would be for us. I got out of the bath and my contractions stayed around 8-9 minutes apart all night.

I was shocked at the power my body had. I used all my brain energy to embrace and welcome each contraction and not sink in fear. Sometimes I failed and allowed the pain and fear to overcome me. But there would come a break. I could refocus and approach the next contraction with a clear and strong mind. Nick was my rock. He would give pressure to my hips each time and he coached me during and between each contraction. We walked together, we kissed, we hugged, and he was my safety.

Seventeen hours had passed. My midwife came to check on me. I was four centimeters dilated. I felt so defeated. Seventeen hours of hard work for only four centimeters? That didn't seem fair. It was then I had a choice. Feel sorry for myself and complain or continue to fight. After a few minutes of sadness and pity, I decided to try something new. My team set up the birth pool and I got in. In the water I was able to melt into each contraction. I could surrender to the power inside my body.

I began to talk to Crosby. "Come out baby. Move down honey. Crosby, sweet boy, we are excited to see you." This calmed me and I remembered there was a purpose and there was a prize at the end. Something changed in the water and I felt in control. Nick whispered, "You are so strong, you CAN do this." He was right. Those words helped more than anything else and came at the right time.

After 30 minutes in the pool, I asked my midwife to check my dilation again. I was eight centimeters. I had dilated four centimeters in half an hour. A few minutes after that, I felt the urge to push. My doctor, midwife, doula, sisters, mom, and Nick were all with me now. I started to push in the water. I was exhausted. My midwife coached my breathing and pushing.

I felt confident and was able to connect with my body. It felt amazing to push. No pain, just power. After a few pushes, Crosby's heart rate dropped and I was quickly moved to my bed. I was hit with fear and panic. My breathing was quick and shallow. My midwife grabbed my shoulders and locked eyes with me.

"Megan! Stop that! You can do this," she shouted.

Oh … right! I needed that reminder. I was in this. I was so close to the finish line. I was capable to birth my child and I could do it with strength and confidence. I pushed through two more contractions and reached down to feel Crosby's head, his face, his little hand resting on his cheek, and before I knew it, my doctor said, "Go ahead, grab your baby, hold your baby."

I had done it.

On November 12th, our precious 7 pound and 2 ounce baby boy was born. My eyes searched for Nick's and we just stared at each other. "We did it," I said. We were lost in this beautiful moment together when we heard our son Crosby's cry for the first time. I was so connected to Nick that I had almost forgotten our baby had been born. We both looked at our baby and were filled with love and excitement and gratitude for this tiny soul that was given to us. Crosby is a beautiful, healthy, strong boy and the perfect addition to our family.

November 13, 2021

Kristen, Hector, and Lilliana

Our birth story started much like our conception story… with a bang. Trevor and I were on our honeymoon in Miami, Florida and had an afternoon quickie to celebrate both our marriage and our first pregnancy with twins. Afterwards, I had persistent cramping. After several hours, it was agreed upon to head to the hospital.

After being admitted to Triage alone because of COVID protocols, I explained my situation and I was hooked up to a contraction monitor to see what was happening, but they never really picked up anything. After about 4 hours of nurses who didn't quite believe me, everyone kicked into gear once my water broke. I was then given my first cervical check ever and was dilated to 2 centimeters.

I was admitted to labor and delivery, where Trevor was able to join me. We spoke to at least 15 different doctors, all giving us new information, like what to expect if I were to deliver right now, resuscitation of premature babies, likelihood of survival, etc. It was so difficult to process, yet I remember it clearly- the body works in mysterious ways to make sure you do everything to save your children. The goal was to keep me at the hospital and delay labor for as long as possible. We were told after waters break, they can keep patients from giving birth "50% of the time." Trevor and I relaxed some and decided that we wouldn't let our families know until we saw where this was going. For the rest of the day, I was confined to bed rest and given a full treatment of magnesium to try and slow labor. I was also given steroids for lung development of premature babies. Aside from that, I was given no pain medication, and no food.

After a relatively calm day, besides my babies refusing to stay on the heart rate monitors for any extended period, everyone agreed to take me off the magnesium and move me to antepartum, where I was to stay for "28 weeks, 30 weeks, and 32 weeks. 32 weeks is the goal!"

I remember laughing with Trevor… because the contractions never stopped, and we told them this. Despite the warnings, the machine wasn't picking them up consistently, so they moved us.

Very quickly, my labor started progressing in antepartum and I drifted off into laborland. The nurse asked me what my pain level was, and I remember contemplating for a while, because if this was early labor, I couldn't possibly be in that much pain. So, I said a level 7, and she looked at me and said, "You're saying 7, but you look like a 10. I can't believe they'd move you down here if you are in labor?"

Trevor and I were also confused, but I knew that things were picking up. Luckily, Trevor had the foresight to keep track of contractions on his phone, and I was having them every 4 to 5 minutes. Once I started throwing up, I knew my cervix was softening and I begged Trevor to get our nurse again. We finally got an OB to come down after a few hours in antepartum, and she asked if she could do a cervical check. I consented and to my horror, she said, "You're still at a 3! This is great news!"

They moved me back to the labor and delivery ward, but at this point, I could barely move, the contractions were coming in so quickly and I had never experienced that type of intense pain ever in my life. I was begging for pain relief at this point because I knew I couldn't do this for weeks. After a moment of screaming, "The little boy is just scratching his fingers nails all over my uterus!" another OB asked if she could check me, and I agreed. Once she was inside me, she huffed very deeply and said, "You're fully dilated," and she ran out of the room and informed every single person on staff. After 36 hours of contractions, my impatiently sweet babies decided they were ready to enter Earthside.

I was then given an ultrasound to see where they were both facing, and they were both still breech. So, Baby A would come vaginally, but Baby B was going to be delivered via c-section. Then, I was swept away in the most dramatic fashion and pushed down the hallway to the OR. My feet were put in the highest stirrups, I couldn't even see my vagina over my grown belly, and they told me to start pushing. I pushed and remembered looking for Trevor, who they locked out of the room. But Baby A was coming, despite only being 25 weeks old. He cried a perfect little puppy cry, and let the world know he was here, arriving at 3:11am. I said hello and cried while they rushed him away.

At some point, the team decided that Baby B could also come vaginally, and they stopped prepping me for surgery. Soon enough, I felt the urge to push after Trevor came in - I just needed a little oxytocin. I pushed and Baby Girl came out, giving us the sweetest little kitten cry and modeling the most beautiful blonde peach fuzz I'd ever seen. She was born 7 minutes after her brother, at 3:18am. She was also rushed away to the NICU and Trevor and I were in shock, but yet so happy.

We had crying babies.

We didn't name Baby Girl B and Baby Boy A for nearly 2 days, but we finally settled on Hector Michael and Liliana Winter. Hector and Liliana had a beautiful ten days in the NICU, enjoying their parent's voices and learning about the world. They both got a bacterial infection that took them away from us too soon, but they were born fighters, and we will forever honor their memories because they made us parents.

Hector Michael Pollom and Liliana Winter Pollom
11.13.21 -11.23.21

November 14, 2021

Brenna and Samuel: A Birth in North Dakota

Our first baby, a boy, was due on November 12, 2021. We had an appointment scheduled with our midwife that day. My parents were staying with us while waiting for his arrival, so they tagged along. Baby and I were in perfect health without a single complication the whole pregnancy. He had dropped pretty low into my pelvis but otherwise seemed very cozy and unlikely to come soon, especially since I was a first-time mom. Our midwife even mentioned that he seemed on the smaller side still and might need a little more time to "cook." Good thing, as she was going to be out of town for the weekend and we would have been so sad for her to miss it!

To my surprise, early the next morning, I woke to some mild contractions as the first heavy snow of the season fell in Grand Forks, North Dakota. Around noon, I went to the bathroom and found I had lost my mucus plug and my water was leaking. Contractions were still very mild but started coming every twenty minutes. I excitedly told my mom and we texted my husband Scott and my dad who had gone out to the store. They brought me back a beautiful bouquet of flowers and some of my favorite snacks. It was still very early but we were so excited it was happening!

We let our midwife know that things had started and to our relief she told us that she would be staying in town because of the poor road conditions from the storm. It was the first time I could say I was grateful for snow in North Dakota! That afternoon, we hunkered down to watch the snow fall while I relaxed with our dogs. My mom and husband cleaned and blew up the birth pool, and my dad prepared food for everyone.

That evening, contractions were coming more frequently, and I started experiencing back labor, which made it difficult to get comfortable. We watched a movie as I worked through them on the birthing ball. I sent my husband to bed so he would have energy for the long day ahead and my mom stayed with me in the living room as I tried to sleep as much as I could while kneeling over pillows we propped up on the couch.

In the early morning, I took a shower and the hot water felt amazing until it ran out. Contractions got much more intense and started requiring all of my attention. I decided I wanted to get in the birth pool and needed more support, so I woke Scott up to start filling it. Contractions were coming about 3-5 minutes apart at this point, so we called our midwife to let her know she'd probably need to come soon. My dad brought buckets of hot water to keep the pool warm when needed and my mom and Scott took turns applying counter pressure, keeping a cool cloth on my head, and bringing a drink to my mouth.

Our midwife arrived soon after the sunrise. Over the next few hours I listened to Hypnobirthing tracks, focused on my breathing, and took tiny naps between contractions. To my surprise, my body started pushing. I had remained very calm and never realized I was in transition.

Our midwife thought it would be helpful for me to move to the toilet for a while. Anything that meant getting out of the water sounded horrible, but I knew I should keep moving. She confirmed she could see his head. My husband told me that he had lots of black hair and encouraged me by reminding me how close we were to meeting our baby. Our midwife's assistant arrived around this time and we decided I should get back in the pool if that's where I wanted to have the baby.

I got back in my favorite position, on my knees leaning over the side of the pool. The first contraction after I got back in, the fetal ejection reflex kicked in and his entire body shot out in front of me. I was in shock until I heard our midwife call out, "Baby! Baby, Brenna! Grab your baby!" With her help, I pulled him up out of the water and onto my chest at 12:55pm. He let out a good strong cry almost immediately and we were all so thankful he was finally here.

We spent the next golden hour in the pool, peacefully getting to know every precious detail of him. He instinctively latched very quickly and nursed for a long time while our dogs peeked over my shoulder, curious about the new, noisy little human in our home. We could tell from the shape of his head that he had come out asynclitic, probably because he had been posterior for most of labor and didn't make his full turn around before I started to push.

The placenta still hadn't emerged, so Scott cut his cord and enjoyed some skin to skin time with him while I delivered it on a stool outside the pool. It felt so amazing to take a shower, get into clean clothes, and snuggle up with my little family after a long day of labor. Our midwife performed his newborn exam at the foot of our bed where he got a perfect bill of health and weighed in at 7 pounds 4 ounces and was 21 inches long. I couldn't have asked for a more perfect Sunday afternoon to welcome our sweet Samuel into the world, surrounded by the love of his parents, grandparents, and incredible birth workers.

November 16, 2021

Paige and Avery

I had been doing so many things to make sure that Avery would be in a good position for birth. That day I had a great leg workout. I did lots of squats and half lunges and was very intentional with my movement and trying to get her engaged in the right position. In the afternoon my two older kids and I went to the park and I walked up and down a grassy hill while they rode bikes. While I made dinner that night, I started having some mild cramping and wondered if it could be the start of labor...

After dinner we went upstairs and I threw the kids in the shower while I attempted to stretch to help with my lower back pain. My little Braxton hicks started feeling more intense and I ended up on my knees hugging my birth ball while my belly hung. My husband, Jonathan, walked in the door and I told him things felt more intense than usual, but I still wasn't convinced it was real labor. He finished up showering the kids and I had maybe two more contractions before I realized this could be it.

I texted my midwife and doula just to let them know something might be happening! Around 7:00pm my midwife asked if my contractions were random and if I was timing any. I sent my midwife a screenshot to show her they were about 2-3 min apart and lasting over a minute already. I remember thinking that surely I was timing wrong, because that was too close together already!

My midwife and doula started to head over to our home. Before my doula arrived, I had a contraction that dropped me to my hands and knees and I instantly felt pushy. I ripped off my bottoms and there was blood. I called for Jonathan telling him I needed him to tell my midwife and doula how I was feeling. My doula told me to put towels and pads down and crawl to the carpet to get on something softer. I ended up on my hands and knees in my bedroom.

My mom showed up and then my doula. The pool was already being filled at this point, but I wasn't allowed in until my midwife got there and she lived a little farther away. I say I "wasn't allowed," but my doula just knew that if I got into the tub at that point, I would have the baby pretty fast and my midwife wouldn't be there. I rode out contractions trying to breathe through them and not push. IT WAS INTENSE!

I was feeling so much tightening and back pain during each contraction. My doula brought me down when I would start to feel scared. I would breathe in and breathe out a very loud and low moan. Jonathan was my rock through them. I wanted his hand just placed on my back and I could hear him whisper to breathe out deeply. When my midwife was pulling up to my house, I got the ok to get in the pool.

It was amazing! My body instantly relaxed in the warm water and the contractions I had in there felt so much more manageable.

I did a few contractions on my knees hanging over the side of the tub. Then I flipped over and rested back on Jonathan. His arms were under my armpits holding me up. I know this was not comfortable for him, but it felt great for me. He didn't complain at all and just did what I needed. By this point my baby was coming down. I focused on my breathing and allowing my tissue to stretch. My body pushed on its own and all I did was breathe. The ring of fire was not that bad and I think being in the water helped a lot. When her head was out, I reached down to feel her while I waited for the next contraction. I could feel her rotating inside me and it was such a weird feeling. At this point we noticed her cord was wrapped around her neck, but I knew that it's completely normal and nothing to worry about. The next contraction started and I felt my body pushing. I used my core and pushed while breathing out, never holding my breath. She came right out!

The sense of relief was amazing, but the feeling of having my baby here was something I can't describe. My midwife unwrapped the cord and I reached and pulled her up to my chest. At that moment I couldn't believe that she was here. It was over. Everything I had prayed about, read about, and hoped for was actually here. I got to experience that birth high I hoped for! It was incredibly healing for me.

My two little ones were sitting behind me on the bed watching and cheering me on the whole time. Avery was born at 8:49pm, so it was only about 2 hours of labor! Delivering the placenta…sucked. If I'm being honest I didn't love that part and I would much rather birth a baby. It took maybe 45 minutes to come out, but once Avery started nursing it helped the process. My older daughter, Emmy, was really excited to cut the cord so she got to do the honor with a little bit of help from her Dad. After that I showered and Jonathan got to do some skin to skin. I got out of the shower and got straight in bed with my little family all snuggled up close to our new baby.

I'm so grateful I decided to have a homebirth. It was the most peaceful and beautiful way to bring a baby into the world.

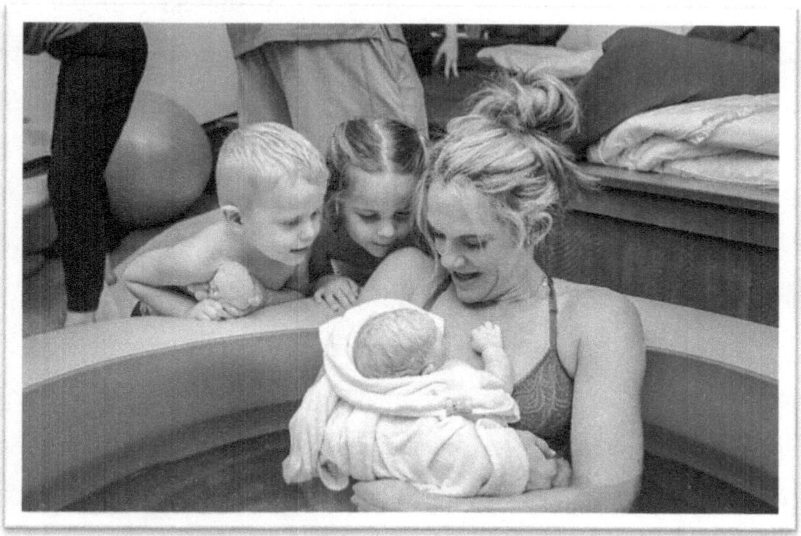

Photo by Danielle Randall
Sunshine Doulas

November 17, 2021

Keerstin and Arrow: A Birth in Missouri

I was induced on November 17, 2021. My swelling was getting out of control and my blood pressure was rising, which was concerning to my OB. She decided it was baby time. Induction was the absolute last thing on my mind, so I was fighting off a panic attack as my husband and I went home to grab our bags and head to the hospital. Once checked in, they gave me Misoprostol to thin my cervix, I ate dinner, and tried to rest. I woke up at 2:45 the next morning to use the restroom and before I sat back down on the bed my water broke. My OB let me labor naturally as long as I could. I was dilated between 7 and 8 centimeters when they put me on Pitocin. My mom had natural births with all five of my siblings, so I remained determined to follow in her footsteps.

Up until this point my pain level was a six during contractions. I got one dose of Fentanyl at the same time they started my Pitocin drip and I proceeded to nap for one hour before waking up to the most intense contractions yet. I labored for another two hours with these contractions. I came to the point of thinking, "I cannot do this another second," and then a few moments later started pushing. Not purposely, my body had taken over and within six pushes my baby was here. It was less than an hour after he was in my arms that I understood how people have multiple kids.

I thought to myself, "That wasn't so bad. I could do that again!"

My next birth, assuming I go into labor naturally, I have full confidence in my ability to birth naturally. It was hands down the most intense and empowering experience of my life.

November 19, 2021

Cora and Baby L

At 38 weeks and 4 days I had contractions all day. By evening, my contractions were intense and I made the call to the babysitter to come get my 2-year-old. My husband and I made our 1½ hour drive to the hospital run by midwives. By the time we got there my contractions had subsided. I allowed them to do a cervical check and was 5 centimeters dilated and 90% effaced. They admitted me and I made my way to my room at 7:00pm. There was no baby by the next morning and at 10:00am I asked for my water to be broken after no progression. After four huge contractions and my daughter's heartbeat dropping and my heart racing more than it should, she was here in my arms. My natural birth in the hospital was such a great experience. The next day we headed home to meet big brother and start our crazy life together.

L was born weighing 7 pounds 2 ounces on November 19, 2021.

November 20, 2021

Carley and Tilly: A Birth in Arizona

Labor started on Friday, November 19th with some bloody show and an increase in nesting urges. I was 41 weeks exactly. Despite this being my eighth baby, I had never gone into labor without natural "induction" help, so I was doubtful things were going to progress on their own. After no noticeable difference in the prodromal labor I had been experiencing for weeks, I went to bed feeling discouraged that it would still be another week. Saturday morning I woke up really overwhelmed and emotional and told my midwife that I was not feeling hopeful things were going to happen without her help. Little did I know, she was confident this was the day that baby was coming.

By the late afternoon I needed to stop thinking about labor, so we went to the property that we were building on and walked around. We were there for about an hour and started heading back to our van when the first REAL contraction hit around 6:30pm. I had to stop and work through it and I felt like maybe, just maybe, this was it. I got in the car and we drove the 20 minute drive home while my contractions started coming every 5-7 minutes. By the time we got home I tried to make myself dinner, but I had no appetite anymore and I just wanted to retreat to my room and be in the quiet as the surges came.

My husband decided to let our midwives know because they both had about a 45-60 minute drive to our house. They arrived around 8:30pm and things were picking up in intensity. I was still doubtful things were going to be quick, even though my hubby was reassuring me that I had to be at least 7 centimeters based on my mood.

Around 9:30 I felt the need to lay down and rest in between contractions, still fully convinced I had a long night of labor ahead. I rested for about half an hour and then by that point the tub was filled and ready for me to get in. I got in around 10:00pm and my baby began to shift down. My midwife heard the change in my moans and said I could push whenever my body signaled it was time. Right around 10:15 the contractions began bringing her down. After a little help with a lip, Tilly was born at 10:29pm. She weighed 10 pounds 11 ounces and was 21.5 inches long. She was perfect in every way.

November 22, 2021

Ali and Ella

I didn't go into labor until 41 weeks and 5 days. I was planning an unmedicated birth in a birth center and I was starting to get very anxious that if I didn't go into labor by 42 weeks, I'd have to transfer to the hospital for an induction. Luckily, after trying many of the natural induction methods (castor oil, spicy foods, intimacy), I went into labor that evening around 11:45pm. The contractions started fast and furious, but throughout the night and early morning, slowed down. My mom, husband, and I all went to the birth center in the morning so the midwives could check on my progress. They recommended I go home to continue laboring and keep them updated as things happened.

We attempted a walk at the mall to help get labor going, but I was so tired, I ended up just taking a nap in a massage chair before heading home. As I labored at home, the contractions continued getting stronger and closer together. I felt all of my contractions in my lower back instead of in my abdomen, which made it extremely difficult to find a comfortable position. Finally, around 8:00pm, I decided I was ready to go to the birth center. Not only did I feel like I was getting far enough into active labor to go in, but I felt like it would help me mentally to go in, so I could feel like I was actually going to have this baby and not just be in labor forever.

We got to the birth center around 8:30pm. The birth center is a small center on the fifth floor of an office building. The midwives came down to greet us on the ground floor. As soon as we walked in, they said, "Okay, Ali, we have some bad news. The elevator isn't working. We have to take the stairs." So, I climbed five flights of stairs in active labor. It took me a long time as I had to keep stopping for breaks, but I had my mom, husband, and the midwives behind me cheering me on the whole time.

We finally made it into my birthing room. I got in the tub right away and the water helped enormously with the back pain. After a long time in the tub, my midwives suggested I get out of the tub and try other positions. I tried getting on all fours on the bed, squatting while holding onto a scarf on the wall, sitting on a birth stool, but finally ended up back in the tub. With every contraction, I felt my body involuntarily pushing. By the time I got to the "pushing phase," I felt like I had already been pushing for hours and was exhausted, but determined.

I pushed for over three hours, half on the bed and half in the tub. I kept reaching down and feeling the top of my baby's head as she was crowning. I vocalized very loudly through each contraction and my midwives kept reminding me to vocalize low and deep to help push the baby out. Finally, at 3:16am on November 22, at 42 weeks exactly, my daughter was born in the water.

She was born "sunny side up" meaning she came out with her face towards the sky instead of towards the ground, which explained my back labor. I also found out later at my 6-week appointment that she came out with her chin lifted up instead of tucked into her chest, which is not an optimal position, and is probably why it was so hard to push her out. My midwife said that it is a very rare position for a baby to be born.

After my baby emerged, the midwife lifted her out of the water and put her in my arms. She had the cord wrapped around her neck and torso. They quickly unwrapped her and then I put her up on my chest. After a few blissful moments, someone asked if it was a boy or a girl. In the excitement of the birth, no one thought to look right away. We looked and excitedly announced that we had a girl! My husband announced her name to the room as we already had our names picked out before the birth.

After getting cleaned up and cared for, we headed home about 5 hours after she was born, ready to begin our next adventure as a new family.

November 22, 2021

Misha and Evie

My first pregnancy was twins. I was living in the Czech Republic and I automatically signed up for a hospital birth. Since Baby B was breech, hospital policy would not allow me to try a vaginal birth and I was wheeled off for a scheduled C-Section. This first birth left me hungry for more and I was determined to do whatever it took to have a VBAC.

When I became pregnant again, I quickly realized that birthing at home would give me the best chance at having a successful VBAC. We moved to California in my second trimester and started interviewing midwives. Not all midwives were willing to provide care for a VBAC mama at home, but I was blessed to find one who trusted me and my body. My pregnancy flew by smoothly and I quickly approached my 40-week due date.

At 41 weeks, I started getting anxious, because in California you are ineligible for a home birth after 42 weeks. At 41+2, hoping to naturally induce labor, I made a Castor oil shake. I couldn't keep it down, so I made a second one around 1:30pm. I laid down to rest, thinking that if I stayed still the Castor oil would do its job. An hour and a half later, I felt the waves coming. They were mild period cramps, but they were coming consistently. I focused on relaxing through each one. This was my first taste of labor and I was excited to finally let my body do what it was designed to do.

After 45 minutes I was resting on my hands and knees, leaning on a pillow. The waves were growing in intensity. With each wave, I focused on relaxing every muscle through my body and surrendered to the power that was flowing through me. My parents picked up the

2.5-year-old twins. Our apartment was silent and dark with only my husband and me.

At 7:30pm my husband laid down to nap so that he would be able to support me later in the night. We both were envisioning a long late-night birth. In the silence, I continued to surrender to the waves that were washing over my body. Hymns were playing in the background and it was a beautiful moment. At 9:00pm I woke up my husband because I needed help relaxing through the intensity. We moaned together and he timed the waves for me. There wasn't any noticeable pattern.

At 10:00 I sat down in our little bathtub. I lost my mucus plug and then went back to our bedroom in the dark. There still wasn't any regular frequency, so I was convinced that I was still in the early phases of labor. At 10:45 I sat on the toilet. Curious to know what was happening, I used my finger to feel my vagina. There was an unmistakable "pop" and water gushed. I had broken my own water. I felt again. There was something hard and fuzzy. I froze in disbelief. Could that be my baby's head? I asked my husband to feel and we were amazed. It had only been 7 hours. We immediately called my midwife and she started heading towards us.

By 11:00, I had the urge to poop. Pushing was imminent. My husband quickly started blowing up the birth pool, while I relaxed in our bathtub. All of a sudden I was intensely starving. I wolfed down two protein bars in between the waves. I leaned into the bathtub and primally yelled as the pressure pushed me to my limit. But my limit kept growing and I was riding those majestic waves with the highest crests. I felt so strong, even though I had no idea what was before me nor how I was going to get through it.

Our baby was crowning. The birth pool was forgotten. I stood up, knees bent and at 11:58pm, my husband caught our baby's head. Moments later, my midwife rushed in and helped catch the rest of her body. Happiness overwhelmed me. My body did it. I wasn't "disabled" from my previous C-Section. My body overcame the odds. As I clutched my sweet baby girl to my chest in our tiny apartment bathroom, I realized that this was the most empowering moment of my life.

November 29, 2021

Kelsea and Arthur

Arthur's birth story starts about 3 weeks before he was born when my prodromal labor started. Every few days I would start having contractions, they would be in a regular pattern, usually about 8 minutes apart for a couple of hours, but would never intensify or speed up past that point. So many times in those weeks we thought, "This is it!" only to stall out and eventually have the contractions stop. This was very mentally challenging and I had to focus on surrender and my faith that this little guy would eventually come out. I had to trust that he would come in his own time when it was right for him. But it was hard!

On Monday, November 29, at 40 weeks and 4 days, I woke up around 3:00am with contractions. They were about the same intensity as the contractions I had been having for weeks, but I had never been woken up by them before. I sat on my birth ball and breathed and timed contractions for about an hour. In this time they grew stronger and closer together until they were 5 minutes apart. I woke my husband up around 4:00am. We called the midwife to check in and she said to let her know when we needed more support or when things started to pick up.

At around 7:00am my doula arrived, and my husband left to take our 4-year-old to school. Contractions were still about 5 minutes apart and increasing in intensity. At this point I had to focus and breathe through the contractions, but was still able to have a conversation in between. I moved to my bedroom, which my husband and doula had prepared, and knelt at the end of my bed with a pillow supporting my upper body – I spent most of my labor in this position. I had so many plans to use my tub, shower, birthing ball and rebozo…but in the moment I only wanted to be in that one spot! Around 7:45 I felt like I needed to stand, so I spent a handful of contractions standing and swaying and felt a noticeable shift in the intensity of the contractions. Around this time my husband returned home and he and my doula timed a few contractions.

They called the midwife at about 8:45am since my contractions were now 3 minutes apart and very intense. I had returned to my kneeling position and my doula helped me to focus on getting through every contraction. I knew that I needed to just take them one at time. I focused on relaxing and deep breathing through each one – trying to relax into the purpose of the contraction and let it do its work. At this point I had to really focus through the intensity. I wasn't aware of much that was happening around me, but I knew things were moving quickly. I kept asking my husband how far away the midwife was. At some point I felt a shift in the contractions. I felt my body bearing down.

Finally, the midwife arrived. She pulled up to our house at 10:06am and my husband ran out to help her carry in her things. As she came in, she heard one of my contractions and realized how close we were. She then flew into action getting everything ready. She checked in with me asking how I was doing and checked on baby. Through all of this, my team was always calm and supporting me through the waves. I felt completely supported and trusted and no one there questioned if I could do this. My midwife let me know that she could feel Arthur's head and that we were so close. I had one overwhelming moment of fear and anxiety and told her that I didn't think I could do this. She lovingly and confidently told me, "You already are, Mama."

It was the most intense experience feeling his head make its way out. I rested shortly and my midwife unwrapped the cord from around Arthur's neck (twice!) and then my body was ready to continue. I had a few more strong contractions and pushed and he was out at 10:20am. Carolyn passed him into my arms and I cried in amazement at this tiny human and what we just accomplished together – it was the best feeling and worth every bit of work! Labor was about 7.5 hours with around 3.5 hours in active labor. Sweet baby Arthur McCurry was 7 pounds, 9 ounces, and 21.5 inches long. I had no tearing, no stitches, and crawled into bed to snuggle with my sweet babe and recover. What a blessing a home birth is! I am forever grateful to my midwives, husband, doula, and nurse who all helped support me through. My body knew exactly what to do.

December

December 1, 2021

Hope and Abel: A Birth in Oklahoma

It's 10:00pm on November 30th. My husband, Jorge, and I are dropping off a few items to our friend Alyssa after spending the day moving. I—being hours shy of 41 weeks pregnant—am wiped, so Alyssa comes out to the car to say goodnight to me and my daughter, Carol Lynn. She leans down near my bump and asks when he or she will be making their appearance. She shrugs and says, "All I heard was three o'clock." With that, we head to our AirBnb and settle in.

It's now 1:14am on December 1st. I'm finally crawling into bed and text my friend, Bree. "Nothing too crazy happening right now," since I only feel soreness from moving.

At 2:57am, I wake up to a massive squeeze and quickly realize my blanket is wet. I figure my waters must have released and I must be in labor. I walk to the bathroom and, at 2:59, another wave comes over me. I wake Jorge and tell him we need to call our team.

Jorge dials Ruth, my midwife, and I dial Alyssa and another friend, Lauren. It's now 3:00am.

I test the fluid I lost with an amnio swab just to see, and it isn't amniotic fluid. The contraction came on so strongly that I peed my pants. I crawl back in bed to rest and go inward. For the next 30 minutes I cuddle Carol Lynn, softly singing along to Housefires. I hear my team gathering in the dining area.

I reach the point where I can no longer stay laying down comfortably, so I make my way out of the room. A big, primal groan leaves my mouth and, baffled, I ask, "Why am I moaning? It's too soon for me to be making these noises." Transition was starting.

I find my place at the head of the supper table. Lauren, Alyssa, and Jorge are trying to fill the pool, but the hot water runs out and I know there won't be time to fill it. I'm going to have this baby standing up, just like I did with Carol Lynn.

Things are getting intense now. The heat is set to 72° for baby and I'm sweating. I've been swaying with Jorge for about an hour and I'm getting to a place where I need to dig deep to remain collected. I grip the table and extend to my tip toes as a wave comes over me.

As Ruth checks on the baby, she exchanges a certain glance with her assistant, Marlita. Baby's decelerations aren't where she'd like them to be for a mother who has only been in labor for ninety minutes. There's a part of my mind that goes to the worst-case scenario, but a stronger part of me determines to trust my body. Birth is an emergence, not an emergency.

Jorge and Marlita are taking turns offering counter pressure and Alyssa is passing me steaming washcloths to hold against my pelvis. Pressure is building, and I'm extending to my tip toes again. I rein it back in, flatten my feet, shake my jaw loose, and let out a moan.

I ask, "Am I shitting myself or is it the baby?!" as I work to exhale.

I holler, "Baby, Baby, Baby!" which is Ruth's cue to get ready to catch.

I yell out, "I'm gonna throw up!" as I lower myself into a squat. The Fetal Ejection Reflex takes over and my baby is caught as my waters break. It's 4:59am and my baby is born "in the veil."

I grab hold of my baby and the first thing I can think is, "Those are some massive baby balls!" In the same moment, I realize we have a son and exclaim, "It's Abel! He's here!"

From there, Lauren transfers a still-asleep Carol Lynn to the couch and I'm helped into bed. After a half hour, my placenta comes away but I'm not bleeding and Abel isn't suckling. Ruth asks if she can "massage" my fundus, and I consent. As she mashes on me, a clot the size and shape of a liver comes out. Ruth and Marlita take turns massaging me, and things are managed just fine without any tinctures or Pitocin needed. Abel begins to nurse and my uterus gets the hint to shrink.

Some time passes and Abel is separated from his placenta, he's weighed and measured — 8 pounds 10 ounces and 21.5 inches of pure brawn and sweetness.

December 2, 2021

Becca and Lillian

I was induced with cervadil and Pitocin due to concerns of possible IUGR at 39 weeks. Induction was far from the natural birth I had envisioned. I was so anxious wondering if my baby would be okay. During my first birth I used nitrous for pain. I was devastated when my hopes for a chance at a natural birth wouldn't happen. The Pitocin made my contractions intense and irregular and when I was checked 2 hours after it was started, I was only dilated 2.5 centimeters.

I felt defeated. Soon my contractions quickly intensified and I didn't realize it but I was transitioning. Thirty minutes after my check, I delivered my daughter in a dimly lit room while my favorite song played, feeling every surge and sensation. It was beautiful and peaceful and unexpected. I've come to realize birth rarely looks like we plan it to. But there is beauty and magic in the unexpected.

December 5, 2021

Amy and Tristan

The night before Tristan was born I was having some light pressure waves, but nothing consistent enough to make me think his birth was imminent. He was already 7 days past his guess date, so I figured he could come at any time. Since I had a long first stage of labor with my daughter, Nekoda, I assumed I'd have enough time to set up my birthing crystal grid and maybe bake a treat for my midwives. Instead, after a late-night comedy binge with my husband, Jason, I woke up at 1:30am (after about 2 hours of sleep) to an intense pressure wave.

I wasn't sure at first if my water broke or if the wave was just so strong that it was compressing my bladder. I spent two waves on the toilet and realized my water had broken and woke Jason up to call our midwives and photographer/doula. While we were waiting for them to arrive, I laid on our bedroom floor and Jason got to work setting up the bed and birth pool in our room. I had been practicing hypnobabies for months, and listened to my tracks on the floor. I remember getting so irritated by the noise of the plastic sheet under the tub that I tried to go deeper into hypnosis than I'd ever gone before just to block it out.

When the midwives arrived, they had to all but force me off the floor and onto my bed. The change in position helped, and so did the hip squeezes my midwife Caitlyn did. Once the pool was filled, I got in it and the hot water was heavenly. I needed a lot of counter pressure on my back, so Jason and our photographer/doula Kaylene took turns pressing on my back during each wave. We found out later that Tristan's head was angled into my right hip.

I was quiet throughout my birthing time except for saying "wave" at the beginning of each one to let someone know I needed counter pressure. We tried a few different positions to help labor Tristan down. I really liked being on my knees laying over the edge of the tub with my head on our bed. I kept visualizing a flower blooming open and moaning "open" through each wave. In between waves, Jason and I tried to rest, and we have some adorable photos of us catnapping during labor.

After about 5 hours or so (it didn't feel that long to me), I felt Tristan move down into my pelvis and engage. My midwives had me put one knee up to give him more room, which helped. We didn't get any photos since my head was down, but my midwives told me I smiled the whole time I was pushing him out. I remember talking to him as I was pushing, telling him we were doing it together and that we would get to meet each other soon. His head came out first and then my waves stopped for 3 minutes, which felt like an eternity. Then I was able to push his body out when the next wave hit. He needed a little help taking his first breath, but our midwives stayed calm, which allowed us to do the same. Tristan Alexander Winney was born December 5, 2021 at 8:33am. He weighed 7 pounds 14 ounces and was 21.25 inches long.

At around 10:30am, Koda came home from being at her dad's, and she and I cut Tristan's cord together. The interesting thing about my body is that I grow extra placental lobes. With Koda there were two, this time with Tristan there were three. There were no complications from it, but it is unique, and I enjoyed watching the midwives look it over and explain it to me and Koda. Tristan's birth was a completely healing and transformative experience. After a traumatic first hospital birth, bringing him Earthside in the comfort and safety of our home was exactly what I needed.

December 6, 2021

Julie and Joaquín Mumia: A Birth in Mexico

The morning of December 5th, I woke up with lower back pain, some nausea, and mild irregular contractions. By nightfall those contractions were consistent and growing stronger. At some point I was unable to sleep through them and began moving around. Just me and the wee stranger inside me, beginning our journey towards each other in the dead of night.

We had moved to a small pueblo in Mexico when I was about 7 months pregnant. Around 8 months we found our midwives: two magical and lovely women who apprenticed under an elder Abuela (grandmother) traditional Mexican partera (midwife).

By 10:00am on December 6th, my midwives arrived. We went outside and I labored with my birth ball in the sunshine near the mango tree, whose branches supported me through several contractions. My mother and mother-in-law prepared broths, cacao and snacks for myself and the team, sustaining us for the long journey ahead.

With no real concept of time, I felt myself drift away from reality, away from the heavy physical realm and into something more ethereal. My awareness drifted in and out, carried by the current of my contractions and breath. I entered the sacred birth sphere. Uninterrupted.

My partner got home from work around 3:00pm and we all made our way inside, stopping what felt like every 10 seconds for a contraction. With my consent, my midwife gently and lovingly checked my dilation and I was pleasantly surprised to hear I was at 5 centimeters. "Halfway there!" they cheered me on.

Baby, whose sex we still didn't know, remained a bit high up in my belly. So we used the Rebozo and several different positions to encourage the descent. For many contractions I was hanging from my partner's neck while each midwife held one leg, suspending me in a kind of mid-air squat. I had a hot shower with my love where I briefly cried and released some emotions. I yoni steamed over coffee. I used the bed, and the wall, and the bodies of my partner and midwives. I'm so grateful to have had all the support and freedom to follow my body's lead.

I remember leaning into the pressure I had been feeling while pushing. I allowed the pressure to be in my body instead of pushing against it. With the next breath I felt my pelvis and lower back expand and open up in a way that shocked me in the moment. And then came the poop. My partner and I knew that this meant baby wasn't far behind.

I wobbled my way to the toilet where, after a few particularly painful contractions, my partner saw that our baby was crowning. So I waddled back to the bed and a few pushes later the head was out. And then the head was back in. And then back out. And then back in. Every time I would automatically relax after a contraction, baby would slip back in. So on the third wave, I made the conscious decision to push all the way through. It was at that moment that I took control of my labor, the moment I became a Mother. The next moment, at 8:37pm, our perfect son was on my chest.

A few minutes later the placenta was born, and finally it was complete relief. The contractions were over at last.

Later on, after cries, kisses, and hot chocolate were had, we did a beautiful cord burning ceremony. I showered, my team cleaned up, and we slept so deeply as our new family constellation of three.

December 9, 2021

Alaina and Alec

At the end of my pregnancy, I had over a month of strong sensations that made me feel like birth could happen on any night. On a few nights I even left my bed and lit candles in my living room, ready to meet my baby. I was so convinced that they would come earlier than 40 weeks, even though neither of my other children had. I had even placed my "bet" on the baby coming at 40 weeks and 1 day. So of course, on that exact night I was woken by contractions that I knew were bringing my baby down to meet me.

I tried to relax in bed for the first hour of labor and then I woke my husband to tell him we would have our baby soon. I moved out to the couch for a while and my husband busied himself with some cleaning and prep work. My mom came and helped to get my boys settled. The older one wanted to stay near - we had discussed him being present at the birth and he was pretty excited, but also apprehensive about the idea. I was feeling the need for a change at that point, and I went to my bedroom to lean over my birth ball and vocalize through the big sensations I was having.

I felt like everything was under control and unfolding the way I had envisioned it. Each of my boys came in and chatted with me briefly and then chose to go out. My husband was giving counter pressure on my lower back and still setting up our bedroom as a birth space when I asked him to go ahead and fill up our bathtub in case I wanted to get in the water.

At that point I thought there must be at least another hour or more of labor and I wanted a break from the intensity. It turns out that the intensity was transition. No sooner had my husband turned the water on, I was yelling for him to be back at my side and desperately trying to communicate what I needed from him as contractions slammed one on top of another. I felt a surge and a pop as my waters broke. I think the moments following that were some of the most intense in my entire life. I knew babe was crowning and my husband confirmed that he could see it.

I was on my knees and wanted something solid in front of me to lean onto and I could not for the life of me figure out and articulate what I wanted. My poor mom offered me the birth ball, a laundry basket, and her own arm, but I'm pretty sure I shoved them away and screamed "I NEED YOU!" at my husband and he dove in front of me.

I was clutching at him and hanging on for dear life as our baby crowned and then I had a moment of calm after the head had been born. Then I was gripped by another incredibly powerful sensation and it was all I could do to guide the head down safely as my sweet boy fell to the towel beneath me and immediately let out a beautiful cry. I felt so stunned. We had a midwife who agreed to partner with us and be a witness, so we video called her so she could see the baby. My mom and my husband helped me get into bed where they brought me bone broth to drink as I held my precious new boy, Alec.

The final 15 minutes of my 3-hour labor were so wild and primal, I still feel shocked by it all. It's an amazing thing to feel your body pushing your baby out with no conscious or intentional action on your part. I chose to go through this pregnancy "alone" after I couldn't find midwifery care that aligned with my needs. I felt very alone at some moments, despite full support from my family. I had assumed that I would feel alone in those birth moments, but I actually felt so connected with my husband, especially at the end while he literally held me up. This was my second unattended birth, but my first intentional freebirth. Sometimes I feel like I know myself much more deeply after each birth, but other times I feel like each just uncovers more mystery and power that I can't understand.

December 12, 2021

Allisan and WillaJean: A Birth in Kansas

I'm an MRI tech and my husband is a nurse. We have a two-year-old daughter, who was born in a hospital. I have PCOS and it was and still is a journey to healing and fertility. In early 2021 I found out we were expecting our second daughter. I saw an OB a couple times and expressed that I was considering having a home birth with a midwife. She warned against it and tried to scare me into thinking my baby would probably die if I chose homebirth. The scare tactics and impersonal care solidified my decision to have a home birth.

I contacted the doula from my first birth, who was now also a student midwife. I met with the midwife she was working under who was 2 hours away. This was the closest midwife that would travel to my area. After meeting with her I knew a home birth was exactly what I wanted and needed.

I had an uneventful pregnancy. I had morning sickness for about 20 weeks. I got Covid at 37 weeks, but recovered quickly. I walked, stretched, ate dates, did spinning babies, drank NORA tea, and visited the chiropractor regularly. My first daughter was born at 41+2, so I wasn't expecting a baby until close to 41 weeks. At the end of my 40th week I decided to try acupuncture to encourage labor because I was in a lot more pain than my previous pregnancy. I went for my first appointment Thursday morning and had super strong contractions during my visit. They faded as soon as it was over though. I went again Friday and Saturday morning. By Saturday afternoon I was feeling discouraged. I took a walk and talked to my baby, telling her it was safe to be born and that I loved her and couldn't wait to meet her when she was ready.

I decided to take my older daughter to the Christmas parade that evening to take my mind off labor. We walked and got pictures with Santa. At midnight that night, I woke up to my water breaking. Contractions started immediately. I let my midwife know they were about 10 minutes apart and I laid back down to rest and prepare my mind. Around 4:00am my contractions were about a minute long and 5 minutes apart, so I called the midwife again and she headed to our house.

The student midwife who attended my first birth as my doula was only 30 minutes away and got there around 5:00am. The midwife got to our house around 6:00am. They said I was progressing well and they set up the birth pool and let me work through contractions. I sat on the yoga ball in my dark bedroom until about 7:00am. At that point they told me I could get in the pool, so I did that. The water felt so amazingly good and gave me a break from contractions for a little bit.

My two-year-old woke up and my mom came to pick her up. My husband sat outside the pool and let me hang on to his arms as I kept working through contractions. I kind of lost sense of time here and I think I was in transition. I know I threw up and I noticed it was getting light outside. I asked the midwife to check me because I was feeling a little pushy. She said I had some cervix left and suggested I try some different positions. Everyone left the room except my husband, and I tried to move around.

The next thing I know my body was really pushing, but I didn't feel like I was making any progress. I think I was fighting my body and the contractions. My midwife reminded me of how I needed to push and suggested moving to a squatting position. I wasn't sure how I'd move at that moment, but I did with some help. As soon as I got vertical I felt my baby come barreling down. I worked hard and pushed for I'm not sure how long. Eventually her head was halfway out. With the next push her head came all the way out. The midwife helped me move into a runner's lunge position and with the next push the baby came out to her hips and got stuck. The midwife pulled her out the rest of the way. WillaJean Kaye was born at 9:57am. She cried immediately and they handed her to me. She was perfect.

I held her until her cord was white and flat and then we cut the cord and I got out of the pool. My contractions had completely stopped, so she gave me a shot of Pitocin and put me on the birth stool. That didn't seem to help so she gave me an herb and my body pushed the placenta right out. I had been bleeding a lot and was super weak and dizzy and on the verge of passing out. They helped me to the couch and wrapped me in a warm blanket with my baby. I got a bag of IV fluids. When I was feeling better, they helped me to the bathroom and I got dressed. Then I snuggled my baby in bed and nursed her.

The midwives did the newborn exam at our bedside. WillaJean weighed 10 pounds and 8 ounces. I had one small first degree tear. Everyone cleaned up and went home. Postpartum recovery was so much better than with my hospital birth.

December 14, 2021

Jodie and Elliot: A Birth in England

I elected to have a c-section this time following a prolonged labour which resulted in a category 1 Emergency Cesarean the first time I gave birth.

We arrived on the maternity ward at 7:00am. After checking myself (and my expressed colostrum!) in, both my partner and I did a rapid covid test which thankfully were negative. At this point I was allocated a bed and was visited by several staff members including the consultant and anaesthetist who would be performing my cesarean. Both made a great effort to put me at ease by speaking to me about what their role was in the surgery and giving me an opportunity to ask any questions.

Then came the long wait to be called to theatre. I had to give my bed to a lady who was having an emergency c-section, and I was moved to a different waiting room. The new room unfortunately only had your classic hospital waiting room chairs. It was not at all comfortable.

Despite this, I think due to the chaos and trauma of my first birth, I could only feel calm during this time. Finally, we went down to theatre in the late afternoon. By this point my partner was a bit nervy so I was talking him down. The prep for the procedure was very organised and calm. My anaesthetist talked to me the whole way through, from helping me up into the bed to the numbing process itself.

The huge difference this time around was that I was 100% lucid. In my previous c-section I had had pain medication during the labour and was generally exhausted from being in labour for 4 days. So it was somewhat bizarre to just be having a conversation with my partner and the anaesthetist, all the while knowing a team of people were performing surgery to birth my baby! Then in no time we heard the faint cries of our baby boy! It seemed like forever between hearing him and him finally being placed on my chest. He was born at 16:10 and weighed 8 pounds and 7 ounces. I couldn't have hoped for a better birth experience!

I had newborn snuggles while I was being stitched up. Once the surgery was finished, I was moved over onto a bed to be taken out to the recovery ward. I asked to be sat up slightly so I could initiate feeding. Unfortunately, as I hadn't eaten since before midnight the previous day, I was quite light-headed by this point and had to be laid back down again!

I was then taken to the recovery ward where I was monitored for around 7 hours before being moved to the normal maternity ward. There are risks with any surgery, but for me this was the best way for my birth to happen. I was very fortunate to not have any complications, just a healthy baby boy!

December 15, 2021
Emma and Levi

I found out I was pregnant when I was 20 years old and living in Tennessee. My pregnancy was amazing from the start, aside from puking all day every day for the first 15 weeks. I felt his kicks very early on and truly enjoyed being pregnant. Everything was perfect at my 20-week ultrasound, but his growth slowed down each week after that. I practiced meditations and affirmations daily and really wanted as few interventions as possible for our birth journey. The talk of induction started around 37 weeks. By 38.5 weeks they told me they really thought it was medically necessary for an induction. We set it up for December 14th - which just so happened to be my birthday!

We got to the hospital around 8:00am to start the induction process. I got a foley bulb catheter placed around 9:00 and I was 2 centimeters dilated when it was inserted. I had slight cramps, but nothing worse than period cramps. I continued my yoga and stretching for a few hours and took a short nap. At 3:00pm I was 5 centimeters dilated and so excited! At this point they decided to up the Pitocin dosage.

I mostly used the yoga ball at this point until I was checked again. My midwives came around 6:00pm, I ate some dinner, and then I was checked again. I was 7 centimeters and couldn't believe it. This was my first birth and I was so proud of how my body was handling it. I had my mom and husband in the room the entire time helping with massages and encouraging me with my affirmations. My contractions picked up a bit, so I tried getting in the birthing tub, but I hated it.

When I was checked again an hour later I was still only 7 centimeters and for the first time I was disappointed and started to falter in my strength. Pitocin can affect the mind and body and at this point it was being pumped through me. At 9:00pm I was progressing and things were getting more intense. I remember asking for laughing gas and then yelling for them to leave. I kept changing my mind back and forth.

It was around 11:00pm when I had a strong urge to push. My midwife had believed I wouldn't be ready to push until closer to 2:00am and didn't feel the need to check me yet. I convinced her to check me and sure enough I was fully dilated. Around 11:30 I started trying a few different positions and breathing techniques to see which one I preferred. After laboring so long with Pitocin, my body really couldn't handle any position other than lying down sideways.

Pushing was very empowering. I would say I actually enjoyed it, as I did most of my labor as well. I had made it the whole way without any pain medication and the relief that it was all ending soon and I would meet our baby was definitely helping. My baby was born at 12:17am on December 15th. I wondered my entire pregnancy what we would name him but as soon as he was born, I knew he was Levi. The biggest lesson I learned from my pregnancy and birth was to trust my body and trust my instincts.

December 18, 2021

Lauren

I went to the hospital around 9:00am on Dec 17th and started my induction sometime around noon. I got a foley balloon inserted and by 7:00pm it had fallen out and I was 5 centimeters dilated. I started having contractions on my own, but they weren't very strong and weren't helping me progress. Around 2:00am they decided to give me a little Pitocin to get things moving. At this point contractions were picking up and getting much stronger. Thankfully it wasn't crazy painful for me yet.

My water broke around 4:00am. I got up and my nurse helped me get changed and then they changed the bed sheets. All of a sudden after I laid back down the pain was unbearable. I was crying and asking them to just get him out! The doctor checked me and said I was still only 7 centimeters so I asked if I could please go on all fours. I rocked back and forth and just kept feeling the urge to push!

I told my doctor I had to push. There was no way I couldn't and I flipped back over. She checked me and I was 10 centimeters! I started pushing, I pushed for 4 minutes (it felt like way longer) and my baby boy was born! The time from my water breaking to my son being born was only 27 minutes! But it was the most painful 27 minutes of my life! I'd 1000% do another birth without pain medication. The recovery was so much better than my first two births with an epidural!

December 19, 2021

Jessie and Andie

I went into labor at 41 weeks 5 days. I lost my insurance at 38 weeks and had already considered a home birth in the future, so I thought why not? My husband was starting a new business and had just moved us 1,600 miles from home. We were saving for a house, so money was tight. I had been practicing hypnobirthing and I think it helped immensely.

My contractions started at 4:00am and within the hour were coming 4-5 minutes apart. After being checked by my midwife, she found I was fully dilated 10 hours later. I had been using the yoga ball, counter pressure, and finally the inflatable tub to manage my pain throughout labor. But I had a feeling something wasn't quite right. I didn't feel the need to push and my back pain was excruciating. I couldn't explain it, but I just felt like something was off. I told my concerns to the midwife but she assured me she could feel the baby was close and that my waters were going to break any minute.

I labored at 10 centimeters for 3 more hours with my contractions coming every 48 seconds instead of the every 2-3 minutes like they had been. I was exhausted with no break to rest. When I was struggling to open my eyes, I knew that if this baby did eventually come, I wouldn't have the energy to push her out. I decided it was time to go to the hospital at 5:00pm. My water wasn't breaking and the midwife just kept telling me, "It will break any minute!" I told her I was done waiting. She said, "I just feel like you're giving up."

Well, that did it. I ignored my husband, who was trying to avoid a car birth, and went past the doula and the midwife and damn near walked out of there naked. When I got to the hospital they checked me and told me I was actually dilated 5 centimeters and my baby was flipped sunny side. I was given an epidural and passed out.

The epidural slowed my contractions down to every 5-8 minutes and my water broke in my sleep. Baby was born with vacuum assistance at 4:30am the next morning weighing 8 pounds and 10 ounces. Throughout my labor at home, I didn't receive much support from my doula, except occasionally hearing her tell me to breathe from the back of the room. My sisters told me later that she was mostly just doing online grocery shopping or texting. My husband did counter-pressure on me the full 13 hours I labored at home, he was exhausted almost as much as I was. My midwife told me later that I must've shut down labor and closed up on the drive to the hospital. I'm not quite sure what I believe, but I will try a natural birth again for my next baby.

December 20, 2021

Cadiey and Atties

It was a cold December afternoon, and I was 40 weeks and 3 days with my second child. I had been having terrible back pain for weeks due to the baby being posterior. My contractions started around noon, slowly but strong. My 15-month-old son was already with his Oma for the night, and my partner was at work. I labored alone and timed my contractions for a couple hours. By the time my partner got home, the contractions had slowed. I still contacted my midwife just to let her know what had been happening. She said it didn't sound like "real labor" but to call if I needed her. I remembered with my first baby I had ongoing "false labor" for weeks.

I ate some pasta and went to sleep around 8:30pm. At midnight, I woke up to pee and had some period like cramping. When I woke up again at 2:30, labor was in full swing. I woke up my boyfriend and let him know I was going to take a bath. With my previous labor being over 18 hours long and ending in a home birth to hospital transfer, I was anxious about calling my midwife too early. I labored in the tub until around 3:00am. Being the butter fingers that I am, I dropped my phone in the water. I gathered myself to wake up my partner. He called our midwife, who said she would be over in one hour.

As my boyfriend started the woodstove, I labored in the bathroom. I would stand, lean against the washer, squat, sit on the toilet, and get on my hands and knees. I nursed my oldest the entire pregnancy and, being away from my son and not pumping that day, I remember my boobs were leaking.

I had terrible back labor. I just kept trying to move and get comfortable. It was almost 4:00am, and blood was dripping down my legs. I laid on my mattress and started to push my bag of water out. My midwife and her assistant arrived as my amniotic sac dangled from between my legs. At this point, I'm not sure if she popped the bag or if it just broke from the pressure. The assistant raced to try and get everything ready. I remember looking into my midwife's eyes and apologizing because I needed to poop. She just laughed, and smiled as if to say, "You are doing great."

I pushed on my hands and knees on the floor and the head emerged. My midwife checked the cord, and it was wrapped twice around his shoulders. I pushed and pushed, but he was stuck! Panic consumed me. I felt like I couldn't breathe deep enough. I didn't remember it being so hard. The assistant suggested that I get up on my knees. It was all a blur. Baby finally slid down gently to the floor. The room was still. I scooped him up and brought him to my chest, sitting back. He wasn't breathing well, so the assistant gave him oxygen with a mask. It took just a couple moments and then he started crying. Relief. I sat back on the mattress in front of the roaring fire, nursing my baby as my midwife stitched up my second degree tear.

Around 4:20am, I delivered my 9 pound, 3 ounce, healthy baby boy. We chose not to find out the gender, but the entire pregnancy we thought it was a girl. We didn't have a name picked out for a boy! After two days, we finally decided on Atlas Llewellyn. We call him Attie. The entire labor was like a run-away train, but I couldn't have been happier. After my midwife left, and my partner fell asleep, I laid there with my son in my arms, watching the sun rise and feeling so in love.

December 23, 2021

Baby Viv: A Birth in Missouri

I am a bedside nurse in Kansas City, Missouri. I was 36 weeks and 5 days pregnant with my first baby when I went into work on December 22nd. It was my last shift before Christmas. At 6:00pm I was about to leave for work when my lower back started cramping. I had multiple bowel movements throughout the day and was thinking I ate something that just didn't agree with me. When I got to work and started my shift, the cramping in my back became more intense and more regular. I still thought it was nothing.

I did my job as usual until around 9:30pm. I was working on my charting at the computer when I noticed the cramps were becoming even more frequent. My charge nurse noticed something was off when I had a cramp while gowning up to go into a patient's room that caused me to pause. Our tech/nurse's aide that night just had her baby a few months prior and said I looked like I may be having contractions. I was in denial and thought it was just a bad poop pain.

I went back to work and the cramps became even more frequent, so I pulled out my phone and started timing them. They were 1 to 3 minutes apart and had been this way for over an hour. By 11:00pm I couldn't focus on work any longer and was forced to face the fact that I need to get checked out. I tried arguing with my charge nurse that I could drive home and have my husband bring me back. That did not go over well, and I called my husband to let him know that I was getting checked and to get the bags and car seat ready. (Our bags were not packed and the car seat was not installed yet. We thought we had at least another week!) My charge nurse said she was going to go get the wheelchair and I tried insisting I could walk. She wasn't going to allow that either.

At midnight I got checked in and hooked up to the monitor. They checked my cervix for the first time and I was already 6 centimeters dilated. I gave my husband and my mom a call and said I would be having the baby soon. It took an hour to get admitted and settled in our room. They were concerned due to my blood pressure readings being elevated as it could be a sign of preeclampsia. I sat on a birthing ball for 10-15 minutes and then anesthesia came in to offer an epidural. I asked to wait a bit to see how far I could go without it. A nurse came back in to check my blood pressure and see how I was managing. I asked for a cervical check and I was at 8.5 centimeters. Then my water broke.

My daughter did not like how fast she was coming, and her heart rate dropped. They had me move into all sorts of positions to try and help my baby's heart rate stabilize. While on my hands and knees, the contractions reached their peak, and I was really feeling the urge to push. I got into pushing position and pushed for about 10-15 minutes total. At 2:10am, my 5 pound 12 ounce Viv arrived. She was so little we needed preemie clothes and she came so fast she never got a cone head!

When my contractions got very intense towards the end of labor, I was starting to rethink that epidural. Looking back now, I am glad I was able to go natural and plan to do the same for future babies as well. My manager and coworkers joke about how they almost had to deliver a baby in our unit.

December 28, 2021

Elise and Rosalyn: A Breech Birth in Canada

I was due with my second daughter on January 4, 2022. When I was 32 weeks, I found out that baby was laying in a breech position. I have a septate uterus so the chances of her flipping were slim. Because I was in the care of a midwife, I had to get referred to an obstetrician since midwife's are not able to deliver breech babies in Canada. I spoke to four OB's who all said I should have a c-section. I had done a lot of research and knew that since this was my second baby, I should be able to deliver her vaginally.

I pressed to get referred to an OB who was known for delivering breech babies vaginally at one of the hospitals. I felt so much better when I was transferred into her care. She tried an ECV, but it was unsuccessful. I still felt optimistic going forward that I was in good hands. I had joint care between my midwife and this OB for two weeks and at 38+6 weeks on December 28th, I woke up at 4:00am feeling a lot of pressure and extremely uncomfortable. I emptied my bowels a few times and tried to go back to sleep, but just tossed and turned trying to get comfortable.

By 5:00am, my husband woke up because I was rolling around so much. I asked him to start a bath for me and hoped it would take some of the pressure off. I got into the bath around 5:30 and within a few minutes I started getting back-to-back contractions. After four intense contractions, I felt an incredible urge to push. Terrified, we called our midwife who listened to one contraction and yelled for my husband to call 911 for an emergency transport. She urged me to use horse lips and breathe through them and to not push.

My husband was on the phone with 911 and explained the situation. The fire trucks arrived a few minutes later and our midwife arrived a few minutes after they did and yelled to the firemen to get a stretcher. It was around 6:00am.

Because the ambulance hadn't arrived yet, there was no stretcher. They got me out of the bath and onto my bed on my hands and knees. My midwife discovered that I was fully dilated and she could see my baby's foot and bum. We quickly discussed that we would need to deliver her at home. She called the hospital and luckily the OB we had been speaking to was on call and stayed on the phone with us. With my next contraction I pushed and my baby's feet and bum were birthed.

Then three emergency services personnel arrived and through the change of atmosphere, my contractions stopped. I tried pushing without a contraction, but couldn't get my baby past her belly button. The OB on the phone was discussing with my midwife whether a maneuver would be necessary when I had another contraction. With this contraction my baby's shoulders and arms were birthed and then her head just popped out! My sweet baby girl born at 6:09am, weighing 7 pounds and 4 ounces. She was a little stunned from the quick delivery. Within 45 seconds, after a quick suctioning, she was crying and placed on my chest. I did not have any tearing and we did not even need to transfer to the hospital after she was born. My midwife completed all of the post-birth exams.

It was a whirlwind, precipitous breech birth with a bit of panic, but I wouldn't have it any other way!

Medical Disclaimer:

This book is not an attempt to provide medical advice. It is intended for informational purposes and to share beautiful stories. Always seek the guidance of your doctor or provider with any questions regarding your own pregnancy and health.